HOW TO LOSE WEIGHT IN YOUR SLEEP

EASY NO DIET WEIGHT LOSS SECRETS TO BE AT YOUR DREAM WEIGHT

DANTE SPENCER MA, CSCS

Copyright 2012 by Dante Spencer
Edited by Marine Spencer

ISBN: 061568646X
ISBN 13: 9780615686462

Follow the author on Twitter @_How2LoseWeight
Like *How to Lose Weight in Your Sleep* on Facebook

"Dante Spencer is one of the healthiest people I know. He maintains an impeccable mindfulness about staying in shape and nutrition. He has an abundance of experience in healthy eating that focuses on nourishment, rather than restricting. Dante is like a one-man support system for people who are pursuing a healthy lifestyle...people whose goals are to eat mindfully, fuel the body with healthy foods, and consciously exercise. You'll be inspired by what Dante has to share with you."

-Paula Abdul, singer-songwriter, dancer, choreographer, actress, TV personality

"I asked Dante what he does to always keep his best body. This book is his answer."

-Gerard Butler, actor, *300*

"Dante Spencer is the intersection of brains meets brawn. That's why, for years, so many Hollywood stars have secretly sought him out. Now, Dante's new book 'How to Lose Weight in Your Sleep' reveals how all of us can turn our body into a fat-burning inferno!"

-Cheryl Woodcock, journalist, *Entertainment Tonight*

"This straightforward 'no nonsense' and somewhat sarcastic book is a brilliant read for anyone interested in health and weight loss."

-Michele Domico, MD

"Dante's body looks like a Greek statue, so if you're going to read a book on fitness and health, it should be this one."

-Karen McCullah, screenwriter, *Legally Blonde*

"This book is informative, funny, and extremely well written and I'll be using Dante's strategies in my own training from now on. I really can't recommend it highly enough."

-Ben Cohen, editor of *The Daily Banter*, contributor to *The Huffington Post*

"In his book Dante encompasses his beautiful spirit, soul, and mind. And seeing the man naked brought me closer to God!"

-Ashlan Gorse, TV personality anchor, *E! Entertainment Television*

"One can never be reminded enough that YOU ARE WORTHY of anything you want in life. This book not only promises to deliver what it says, it delivers whether you're sleeping or awake!"

-Jimmy Demers, singer-songwriter, contributor to *The Huffington Post*

"Believing in yourself is the first step. The second is to read this book – it will teach you, guide you, and help you to reach your goals. This book is all the food for the soul you need!"

-Didiayer Snyder, TV personality, *OWN Oprah Winfrey Network*

"From my studies in spiritual psychology, I can attest that in his book Dante clearly understands how the mind affects the body and your ability to lose weight. So there's that and the fact that he is a living, breathing, walking example of what he preaches."

-Lesley Robins, MA, producer *E! News*

"Lose weight in your sleep?? Sounds too good to be true. But, Dante knows what he is talking about. His research is solid and his approach works. Now, if he could tell us how to get rich in our sleep…"

-Alec Musser, fitness model

"Dante Spencer crafts a user-friendly guideline for practical and sustainable fitness using applied kinesiology methods. In addition, he skillfully maintains the integrity of research based practices in movement."

-Carly Marino, MS, exercise physiologist

"Dante has personally helped me drop a significant amount of weight. When it comes to losing weight and getting your best body he knows his stuff. The bottom line is what he shares with you in this book works. "

-Paul Despain, former client

"I wish I read this book ten years ago! 'How to Lose Weight in Your Sleep' is like a health and wellness bible for optimum fitness. In it, Dante Spencer masterfully integrates the three most important aspects of our living: mind, body and spirit. If you are ready for a life change, then you are ready for this book!"

-Jessica Spencer, author of *Rose Colored Glasses,* *Clear Colored Eyes,* radio host

This book is dedicated to my beautiful wife Marine.
Without her, none of this would have been possible.
She is my muse, my guide, my twin flame.
Je t'aime.

TABLE OF CONTENTS

PREFACE

What in the heck gives me the authority to write a book about how to lose weight? Well, I grew up eating poorly like a lot of us. My mom, my stepdad, my sister, and I ate a lot of junk food, microwave dinners, and had fast food almost every week. However, every couple months, my sister and I would visit my father for the weekend. He did natural amateur bodybuilding contests, and also was a personal trainer on the side. He would send me home with stacks and stacks of fitness, health, and exercise magazines. I specifically remember looking at the fitness models on the covers, and saying to myself, "I could never look that good. Those guys are just blessed with good genetics, aren't they?" So even though I wasn't implementing those things I was reading at such an early age, they were slowly being programmed into my head. Finally when I was sixteen, I began to make changes to my health and exercise lifestyle. I had an overwhelmingly strong desire to learn any and everything I possibly could about fitness and nutrition. I had my dad teach me everything he knew. I started studying physiology, and became a personal trainer while I was still in high school. At UCSD (University of

California at San Diego), I minored in biology with an emphasis in nutrition. I ended up being a TA (Teacher's Assistant for the professor) of Human Nutrition. I taught my own discussion class once a week, and had office hours for students to come by and ask me questions about nutrition. I also got the best personal training certifications that were out there: NASM (National Academy of Sports Medicine), APEX (certified nutritionist), CSCS (Certified Strength and Conditioning Specialist from the National Strength and Conditioning Association, NSCA). Soon after, I got a job as a nutritionist and was able to train and implement personal nutrition programs for my clients. I worked with bodybuilders, fitness models, athletes, scientists, doctors, military personnel, disabled people, adolescents as well as the elderly. Meanwhile, I was doing experimentations on myself by eating all different types of foods in all different types of ways, to see what worked and what didn't work in achieving my health and fitness goals. My little personal moment of glory was the first time I found myself on the cover of a major fitness magazine, something I once thought was impossible. Later on, I moved over to the non-physical side and got my master's degree in Spiritual Psychology at USM (University of Santa Monica). Here was a whole new world in which I learned how much our deep emotional issues affect the way we think, and yes... the way we look. I came full circle with knowledge of the body being completed with knowledge of the mind, and saw how much they were related and how they could be put together to work in unison.

So here I was with over fifteen years of hands-on experience feeling a little frustrated because I was only able to help one person at a time. With all the knowledge I had gained over the years, I wanted to help people lose weight on a large scale (no pun intended). That is why I finally decided to write this book, in an effort to help and give this information to as many people as possible, so that all of you could finally have the body you've always dreamed of.

INTRODUCTION

Oh God... not another weight loss book! I'm so sick of hearing about another weight loss, health, or nutrition book written by a doctor or Ph.D. who has a body that nobody wants to have. I'm tired of reading all the crap out there that either doesn't work, that's hard to do, or is a quick fix to lose weight in which you will inevitably gain all the weight back when you stop. It's so confusing in today's world with so many fitness, health, and nutrition magazines, Internet articles, new diet fads, so-called experts, etc. This person says this, that person says that. They say you should eat this way, but not that way. Then you turn around, and you read something that says the complete opposite. You're not sure what kinds of foods you should eat, which ones you should avoid, when you should eat, and how much. On top of that, how and when you should exercise. With all this contradicting and confusing information, you just want to give up and say it's no use. So here you are now, still not happy with the way your body looks, buying another weight loss book with a catchy title. Deep down you don't want to accept that this is the way you are, and that this is the way your body will always be. You no longer want to justify the way you look by telling yourself that there are more important things in life to worry about - job, family, etc. If you're going to live, which you are, why not do it right? Why not do it feeling good and looking good? It's *your* body, it's *your* life, it's *your* choice. How much more beneficial will you be to yourself, to your family, and to your job, feeling good and looking good? How much better of a person will you be with more confidence and more self-esteem? Don't you think that you being at your best will inspire people to be at their best?

Have you seen the movie *300*, the blockbuster that had all those Spartan men with amazing bodies? Gerard Butler, who's a friend of mine, was the main character King Leonidas, and he probably had the best body out of all the Spartans. He worked his butt off dieting and training twice a day for four months prior to the start of shooting the film, and continued to work out and diet heavily until the end of shooting. Cut to a year and a half later, I was visiting Gerard, and I remember during lunch he asked me, "How do you do it? How do you keep your body looking that way all the time?" And I said, "Well, Gerry, you know how to do it. Look at your body for *300*." And he said, "Well that was for a movie. I don't know how to maintain it looking like that all the time. That's why I'm asking you." Well, this book is my answer to Gerard and anybody in the world who is wondering how to get their best body and keep it. This book is the result of well over 10,000 hours of working hard, studying, researching, experimenting on myself, and applying on others to finally know what works and what doesn't work. This is my own personal purging of all the information that is in my head and in my soul. I'm giving it to you so that you no longer have to go on these crazy temporary health kicks. This book is not about a diet. Diets... People always say, "I'm going on a diet." And then what? No one says, "I'm going on a diet... for the rest of my life." What they should really say is, "I'm going on a temporary diet to lose weight, and then of course, I'm going back to the way I was eating before, and I'm going to gain all the weight back. And because of that, I'm going to get depressed and gain even more weight. Then, I'm going to wait around for the next new diet craze, and do it all over again." People always go on a diet as a short-term thing, and that's why their weight loss will always be short-term. Plus, when you think of a diet you think of restriction, in other words, you don't have all the freedom you want. Now, if you're reading this book for a diet that's short-term and restrictive, then you're reading the wrong book. *This book is about a permanent lifestyle change.* The kind of lifestyle where you lose weight in your sleep, have more energy, look younger, and live a happier and longer life.

Now you're probably wondering, "How am I going to do all this? How am I going to lose weight in my sleep?" Well, I've organized this book into five simple chapters, that when you follow... magic happens. The first chapter is on Metabolism and it explains how this fat burning machine works. It also talks about the myths and facts about it, and teaches you how to train and reset it so that it speeds up and burns fat in your sleep. The Nutrition chapter teaches you how to eat properly, and gives you the formula that will help you find the specific amount of food you should be eating to be at your dream weight. The Exercise chapter provides a simple overview of the minimal amount of exercise you need to do to burn fat and have your body looking lean and toned. The Psychology chapter will help you identify and deal with any mental blocks you may not be aware of that can be keeping you from losing weight. And finally, the Detox chapter will show you the importance of doing cleanses in order to flush out the toxins that can be slowing down your metabolism.

This book is all you'll ever need to know. If you apply everything that's in here, you are going to put your body in a situation where it actually burns its own fat in your sleep. That's when you'll start to lose weight while you're dreaming away, rising and shining each morning with a new body.

CHAPTER 1

THE METABOLISM: YOUR FAT BURNING MACHINE

I want to start off this book with a chapter on Metabolism because it is the single most important thing that is going to change for you. The secret of this book lies in speeding up your metabolism as fast as it can be, so that when you go to bed, your body will start to burn its own fat for energy. And, as you got from the title, that's what this book is all about: losing weight in your sleep.

What's up with your metabolism?

Your metabolism is the engine of your body that burns food for energy. What you may not know is that when you put your metabolism in the appropriate condition, it will naturally burn your own body fat for energy. So depending on the circumstances you put it in, your metabolism can be fast – lose fat easily – or slow – gain fat easily. If you're reading this book, most likely you have conditioned your metabolism to be s-l-o-w, which means your body has a tendency to store a lot of fat. That is not a bad thing. It's just that the look of that probably doesn't agree with you, you agree?

What exactly is this fat stuff?

Fat is just *stored energy for later*. There is absolutely nothing wrong with it. Maybe your body has had, up until this point, a lot of stored energy on it. Again, it's not a bad thing because as you will see it has had a *reason* for doing that. And if you no longer give it that reason, then it won't.

Food is energy and nutrients, and the body needs energy and nutrients in order to survive. Food is broken down in the body into sugar, and the body uses sugar for energy. If the body goes long periods of time without food, then blood sugar levels drop, and that signals to the metabolism to slow down. Then, when the body finally gets food, it's going to store as much of it as possible for *survival purposes*. So a slow metabolism will tend to store a lot of body fat. If you were stranded on a desert island with only a small amount of food to last, would you want your metabolism to be slow or fast? Think about it. This brilliant engine knows what to do for survival purposes based on the environment or condition it is put in. It wants to live, so if it has limited food, then it is going to slow down as much as possible, and try to store as much food as it can for later. And what is it called when your body stores food for later? FAT. See fat isn't bad. It's just the body's way of storing energy. Let me ask you another question so we're clear. Who is going to starve to death first on that stranded desert island, a skinny guy with a shredded six-pack or a fat guy? I don't know about you, but I'd put my money on the fat guy surviving longer. The fat guy's fat (also called adipose tissue) will be used on that stranded island for energy to think, to walk, to hunt, to talk... Okay maybe not to talk if there's no one else on the island. A fat guy's body is actually brilliantly effective and efficient solely based on the condition it is put in. So don't judge your body or other people's body as being fat, it's just been in survival mode.

However, none of us are stranded on a desert island with only a small amount of food to last. We have grocery stores on every corner, cupboards and refrigerators filled with food. So since none of us are in any danger of starving to death or have any reason to be in survival mode, I'm going to show you how to make your metabolism fast again, how it's actually made and designed to run from the beginning.

The proof is in the baby pudding

Babies! Remember we were all one of these little guys? Let me ask you a question, something you may have never thought about. How often do babies eat? *Babies eat every 2-3 hours.* We came into this world as these perfect little beings with the eating schedule to have the best and fastest metabolism. Over the course of life, most of us have journeyed away from this, which only means that we have slowed our metabolism, which only means that we store more body fat than we need... and want. Babies are hungry every 2-3 hours. Now look at your mother's breasts (not literally). Nature has designed them to be ready to feed every 2-3 hours. Is that just a coincidence that babies are ready to eat every 2-3 hours, and that mother's breasts are ready to feed them every 2-3 hours? If that doesn't obviously tell us how our bodies are ideally designed to eat, then what does? What other evidence do we need to show us how the human body should be nourished than looking at how we naturally eat and are fed from the moment we come into this world?

Eat small meals every 3 hours... or be fat

Our body only needs a small amount of food every 3 hours to maintain blood sugar levels in order to perform all the millions of functions that keep it alive, and keep it going – from thinking, to breathing, to talking, to walking, to being frustrated with how we look. Eating small meals every 3 hours is the key to having a fast metabolism, and consequently losing weight. Remember, by eating every 3 hours you are maintaining your blood sugar levels, so they never drop. When your blood sugar levels drop from going a long time without eating, it tells your metabolism to slow down, and the body goes into fat storage mode when you eat next. But when the body gets food every 3 hours, it doesn't have a reason to store fat and never gets into that fat storage survival mode. In the normal waking state, eating every 3 hours ends up being five small meals a day (e.g. 7am, 10am, 1pm, 4pm, and 7pm). But if you happen to wake up late and go to bed early one day, then it may only be four meals. So don't worry so much about the number of meals, just focus on eating every 3 hours.

Their fat kept them alive

Besides us current Americans, the only known and recorded obese people in history were a specific tribe of indigenous people. Why were they so fat? Was it because they got the munchies after smoking the peace pipe? No. It was because these people would trek for days without eating, and then when they would arrive at a temporary destination with food, they would gorge and stuff themselves. They did this because they were starving, and they knew they had to travel again for *days* without food. What happened is that their body efficiently started to develop huge fat stores. The fat cells began to increase in number and in size so that they could hold as much stored energy as possible. This was and is strictly for survival purposes. They didn't have mirrors and *Indigenous Cosmo* and *Shape Magazine* hadn't come out yet. These people were just surviving, and their bodies were very effective at it.

Skinny people eat five times a day

When I was a personal trainer before I got certified as a nutritionist, there was an initial set of questions the gym made us ask our clients. The answers to one specific question used to always shock the heck out of me. The question was, "How many meals a day do you eat?" And I'm not kidding, the more overweight the person was the fewer meals they ate, and the thinner the person was the more meals they ate. It was incredible for me to hear this in the beginning. I thought all these overweight people were totally lying about how few meals they ate. But then what about these skinny people? Why would they lie about how many meals they ate? This is the first time it really hit me. I could see how eating many small meals throughout the day – versus two big ones – made a huge difference in the way the body looks. It was so intriguing that I started to guess how many meals the person ate based on how they looked, and I got incredibly good at it. An overweight person would sit down in front of me, and I would say, "So you eat about two meals a day right?" And they would say, "Wow... how did you know that?" I would even guess with the skinny people. A lot of times they were unaware and did it naturally. "So what do you eat? About five meals a day?" They would say, "Hmm... I don't even really count. Let me see. Yeah, about five meals a day. How did you know that?" And I would just smile. This is the biggest unkept secret that most people trying to lose weight don't know about. Most people would think that the more meals you eat, the fatter you will be, and that the fewer meals you eat, the skinnier you will be. But as you now know from reading this, it's just not true.

One large meal a day equals one large butt everyday

Look at sumo wrestlers, known as the biggest and fattest human beings that walk (or pound) the Earth. Guess how many meals they eat a day? *One!* Yes, sumo wrestlers only eat once a day. And this isn't a little salad with dressing on the side, it's one huge gigantic meal! It's actually not even a meal, it's a gosh darn feast! So if you want to look like a sumo, then eat like a sumo.

Size matters

Think of your metabolism as a fire, and think of food as the wood you put on the fire. What's going to happen if you put a huge log on the fire? It's going to slowly burn for many hours, just sitting there. Now, what happens if you just put a few twigs on the fire? They're going to burn up quickly. This is exactly what you want to do with your metabolism. You want to eat small meals (like putting some sticks on the fire) so that your metabolism (the fire) burns them up quickly.

Be hungry every 3 hours

This is the trick! You don't want to just eat every 3 hours, you want to *be hungry* every 3 hours! I've had people who didn't fully get this, and they would tell me, "I feel like I'm eating too much and stuffing myself every 3 hours." And I would say, "Well, guess what? You are! You're eating too much per meal."

We are so conditioned to thinking that a *meal* has to be this big production. It can be as simple as a nutrition bar or a piece of fruit. It doesn't have to be big; it just has to be something. Let's move away from the mentality of large meals and small snacks. Call them *sneals*, or *macks*, or whatever you like. You just want them to be equal to each other so your metabolism can do its job, and doesn't have to guess how much food it may be getting each time. Again, it's just maintaining blood sugar levels, which communicates to your metabolism that it has no reason to slow down and start storing fat. Do you think sumo wrestlers are hungry 3 hours after they eat their feast? So again, you don't just want to eat every 3 hours, you want your body to *be hungry* every 3 hours, and that simply comes from not eating too much each meal. If you are not hungry 3 hours after eating, then you ate too much. In the next chapter, we'll go into the specific amount of calories you should have, but this is a great way to gage, especially if you don't want to be a calorie counter. So when you are about to eat, ask yourself, *"Am I going to be hungry again in 3 hours?"* That will answer all your questions about how much you should be eating.

You're not the size of King Kong

Generally speaking, your two hands cupped together are about the size of 3/4 of your stomach. When you eat, you only want to fill up 3/4 of your stomach, so that you have 1/4 left for digestive juices to come in and begin the digestion process. This is why it's so hard to digest when you're stuffed, because you've filled your stomach completely up. So no more than two cupped hands worth of food per meal. And unless you're King Kong, you don't have hands big enough to fit a big cheeseburger with large fries and a large soda.

Come and get it!

You know those iron triangle dinner bells that are hung on the porch of western houses? When dinner is ready, the mom rings it, and it alarms everybody that it is time to eat. Well, guess what? The great Mother Nature has gifted us with a personal biological alarm inside of us. And it's called... wait for it... wait for it... *the stomach growl!* Can you believe that this priceless alarm clock, that has been given to us for free, has been overlooked by everyone as being just this annoying thing? It's the greatest gift we have to help us get the body we want. Now what exactly is the stomach growl? The stomach growl is a wave of muscle contractions that occurs around two hours after the stomach is empty. A signal is then sent to the brain that in return signals the digestive muscles to get ready for another round of food. The rumbling and gurgling sounds are caused by the digestive system that is preparing to 'eat' again. The warm sensation in the stomach that may be present as well is due to the release of acids and other digestive fluids necessary for the breakdown of food for the digestion process. So the stomach growl actually is this brilliant built-in alarm system that alerts us when the body is ready to eat again. How could we ask for anything better than a noise that emits from the stomach when it is time to eat? In order to train your metabolism to lose weight in your sleep, you want your stomach to lightly growl or have a warm sensation in your stomach like it's about to growl, every 3 hours. This means that you ate just the right amount for your stomach to digest and empty, and then start it all over again. If your stomach doesn't growl or you don't have that warm sensation like it's about to growl, then you ate too much. End of story. Now it's time for you to adjust. The adjustment would be just to eat a little less next time, so that your stomach will growl or feel like it's going to growl 3 hours later. If your stomach growls before 3 hours are up, then you ate too little. So the adjustment would be to eat a little more next time.

Now, if you have a negative association with the stomach growl being a bad thing, you need to understand that there are basically two types of hunger that are completely different from each other. Most people are accustomed to the first one that occurs when you go hours and hours and hours without eating any food, which makes your blood sugar levels go extremely low, creating a weakened, famished state of low energy with heavy hunger pangs. This type of hunger leads to a desperate need to have any type of food quickly without any judgment or consideration of how healthy it is. And the justification for eating bad at this point is, "I haven't eaten all day." Sound familiar? Remember, this is the recipe for gaining weight. The second type of hunger I am talking about here is having that light grumble or warm sensation in your stomach (even though you have eaten 3 hours prior) to tell you that it's time to eat another light meal to keep the fat burning engine going. You will fall in love with hearing your stomach growl or feeling like it's about to growl because you will know it means your body is in dream weight mode and your metabolism is lightening fast. Imagine the kids' faces in the country yard when they hear the triangle bell ring. They smile, drop what they are doing, and run for the house. It's a great thing, it's time to eat! This is what the stomach growl I'm talking about is.

Don't mistake thirst for hunger

If you feel kind of hungry before your 3 hours are up even though you've had the right amount of food, then it just means you're thirsty. So drink water. One of the main things you need to know about your body in regards to water is that you have a thirst mechanism in the brain. This thirst mechanism is really close to the hunger mechanism, and it is weak. A lot of the time we mistake being hungry for being thirsty. The majority of us walk around in a constant state of dehydration. So most of the time when you think you are hungry, you are really just thirsty. Keep water handy and available at all times. Always remember that true hunger has a sensation that you'll feel in the stomach.

The fat burning icing on the cake

Here is one of the biggest secrets to lose weight in your sleep: *do not eat 3 hours before you go to bed!* That's it! That's the icing on the cake. Here is what happens if and only if you've been eating your smaller meals every 3 hours consistently during the day. It's time to go to bed, and it's been 3 hours since your last meal. Your body is ready to eat again, but instead you go to bed. And what will happen is that your body will actually use its own fat as your next meal. So when you are dreaming away in the middle of the night, your body is wildly at work using its own fat for energy. It's like your body is doing its own liposuction while you're dreaming about Brad or Angelina – minus the kids. If you're really hungry at that time, drink water. Water is a natural appetite suppressant. When you drink water and fill up your stomach, the receptors of your stomach send a signal up to the brain saying that you are full, and that's what gives you a feeling of fullness. This is great to always know if you tend to eat too much or want to eat before your 3 hours are up. If you drink water to give yourself that full feeling, and go to bed instead of eating, your body will literally eat its own fat in your sleep. Your fat will begin to melt away. In no time, you will have the body you have always dreamed of. You will have the body that you deserve. And this, my dear friend, is the truth.

Eating breakfast is for champions

When I used to run nutrition programs on people, a majority of those who needed to lose weight didn't eat breakfast. They would get up, hustle around, grab coffee, and head to work. They wouldn't eat their first meal until around lunchtime. Think about it, if they ate dinner around 6pm and were not eating again until around 12pm the next day, that's eighteen hours without eating food. Eighteen hours without the body having any fuel or nutrients. As you know by now, their body is in survival mode and has slowed down its metabolism to bare minimum. And when it eats, it's going to store everything. Wouldn't you, if you were a body and didn't get fuel and nutrients for eighteen hours? Especially if you came into this world getting fuel and nutrients from your mother every 2-3 hours. So in order to lose weight, I had my clients start to eat a small breakfast. Not pancakes and butter or doughnuts, but a healthy, light breakfast like egg whites and toast, or high fiber cereal, or oatmeal, or a smoothie, or a bar, or yogurt, or just some fruit, whatever, just something sensible. Guess what every single one of them who wasn't eating breakfast before said? "When I eat breakfast, I'm like hungry again a few hours later." See, this is what we are talking about. This is exactly what you want! They had thought this was a bad thing, but this is exactly what they needed in order to start training their body to lose weight in their sleep. By having a small breakfast in the morning, you jump-start your metabolism. It's like telling your metabolism, "Get ready because you're going to start going really fast." *Don't skip breakfast or any other meals*, unless you want to skip swimsuit season.

Give two shits if you care

Tracking your bowel movements is a good way to know how fast your metabolism is. It may not sound sexy, but the more often you go, the faster your metabolism is. A healthy person should have at least two bowel movements a day[1]. In my experience as a health professional, the people with the slowest metabolism (thus being heavily overweight) ate two meals a day and had a bowel movement every other day.

Can't blame your genes for not fitting in your jeans

Take identical twin ladies who need to lose a lot of weight. They have the same genetics and eat the same way. Most likely, if they are overweight, they eat two meals a day – a big lunch and a big dinner. Say you take one twin and keep her eating the same way, while her identical twin breaks up the same quantity of food into five meals a day. If you did nothing else but observe, you would see that the twin who started eating five meals a day would have her metabolism start to speed up, and she would begin to shed the fat off. Her body would know it's no longer in survival mode and it wouldn't need to store fat like it did before. One twin would lose her body fat and the other would keep it.

I use this twin example because people like to think that they are how they are because of their genetics. "I'm genetically doomed!" I'm sure you've heard people talk like this. Heck... maybe this has been your excuse. "Why should I even try, it's obvious that I just have bad genetics. Look at my mom... she's

---

1 National Academy of Sports Medicine, *NASM Essentials of Personal Fitness*, June 2011.

fat!" Some studies say that if one of your parents is obese, you have a 50% chance to become obese. And if both of your parents are obese, it's increased to 80%.[2] So from these studies, people just made a grand conclusion that obesity is a genetic factor. However, what they didn't take into consideration was that kids do what their parents do while growing up in the same household, consciously and subconsciously. If the parents are active, then there's a good chance that their kids will be active. If the parents eat healthy, then there's a good chance that the kids will eat healthy. Last time I checked, kids don't provide the food for the household, parents do. When was the last time you saw kids doing the grocery shopping for the family? My point is that parents set the example, kids follow. These studies only mean that 50% *choose* to live the same lifestyle as their parents in their adult life, and the other 50% *choose to* live a different lifestyle – a healthier one. Which one do you want to choose?

Bulimia & Anorexia

Being bulimic or anorexic is an extreme state for your body that has almost compromised its survival. So yes, it's going to take a minute to get back adjusted. Regardless of what you may have read or been told, *you cannot permanently damage or ruin your metabolism*. Even if you used to be bulimic or anorexic, your metabolism can be retrained to be fast and

---

2 American Academy of Child and Adolescent Psychiatry, *Facts for families*, March 2011.

healthy again. Neal Spruce, chairman of the board for the National Academy of Sports Medicine writes, "Your metabolism is not damageable. Take home message: never blame failure on metabolism, no matter what anyone tells you!"[3]

Getting adjusted to your new lifestyle

In the beginning, getting used to eating smaller meals is going to be an adjustment, but your body will adapt within a couple of weeks. At first, you may eat too much at breakfast so that when 3 hours are up your stomach doesn't feel like it wants to growl. It's okay, you just need to adjust and eat fewer calories for your next meal. If your stomach growls before 3 hours are up, then you just ate too little and a slight adjustment is needed. Play with this 3-hour thing and you'll get it right. Make a game out of it. It's pretty fun to play a game that makes you lose weight in your sleep.

People, friends, and family are going to say stuff about how you are eating like, "Why are you eating so little?" or "You are going to starve to death only eating half a sandwich." All you have to do is smile and say, "Yes, I know it seems like I'm eating very little, but I'm eating every 3 hours. My energy levels are high throughout the day, and I'm losing weight in my sleep. You should try." I don't know what mother, grandmother, or friend would have against that. You will actually inspire them,

3 Neal Spruce, *Fact or Fiction: Starvation Mode and Fast Metabolisms*, June 25, 2009.

and it will only be a matter of time before they start to see the physical change happening to you.

We all want to have our personal best body. If you are reading this, chances are that you don't. *Do what's exactly written in this chapter*. Even if you ripped out the pages of the rest of this book and only followed this chapter, you would recondition and reset your metabolism to how it's designed and supposed to be, and you would still lose more weight than you ever dreamed of... while you're dreaming.

"Insanity is doing the same thing over and over again and expecting different results."

-Albert Einstein

A FEW TIPS

Water – Always carry water with you wherever you go. Have a couple non-toxic (BPA-free) plastic bottles, stainless steel, or glass bottles in your car, at work, in your refrigerator, in the bedroom, etc., at all times. The more hydrated you are, the less you will feel the need and desire to overeat.

Snacks – Always carry some sort of quick-to-eat food with you. Always! It can be any sort of meal replacement bar, trail mix, apple, etc. Have it handy at all times in your purse, briefcase, car, or in your desk at work. Plan ahead, so when you get really busy and don't have time to eat, you'll never have an excuse. I just timed myself on how long it took to unwrap and eat a nutrition bar, and it took me about two minutes. And I'm a slow eater. So there's really no excuse. You can eat it in the bathroom, in the car, or on the way to a meeting.

Timer – Set a timer to go off every three hours. (Make sure to set it right *after* you finish eating). I have my timer on my iPhone set to countdown from 3 hours and every time I finish eating I just click my clock icon, hit start, and in 3 hours my little alarm will go off. This is a huge help for me, it takes out all the guesswork in my busy schedule, and I always know exactly when I'm supposed to eat.

THE RECAP

- Eat breakfast in the morning to jump-start your metabolism
- Eat small meals every 3 hours
- Be hungry every 3 hours to make your stomach growl or have that sensation like it's about to growl
- Don't eat more than your two hands cupped together
- Drink water when you feel hungry, you're most likely dehydrated
- Don't eat 3 hours before you go to bed

CHAPTER 2

NUTRITION 101

About fourteen years ago, a shocking thing occurred that would change my opinion of doctors and nutrition forever. I had recently become certified as a nutritionist and was running nutrition programs on clients as well as training them. This one day, I had a scheduled appointment for one of the chief heart surgeons in Southern California to come in as my client for a nutrition plan. She had been written up in the newspapers as the go-to doctor for heart surgery, and she even taught part-time at medical schools to future heart surgeons. I have to admit I was pretty nervous that day. What could I teach any doctor – let alone a premiere heart surgeon – anything that they didn't already know about nutrition? At that point I had been studying nutrition for many years, but that was nothing compared to the amount of school that this heart surgeon had gone through to get to the pinnacle of her career. At first, I had to ask her a bunch of questions about her eating patterns, what kind of foods she ate, her goals, etc. Then came the part I was dreading: the mini-class on nutrition. Prior to this, I prided myself on this 'Me the teacher, my client the student part.' Today was a little different. I was supposed to give my little nutrition lecture to a profound heart surgeon who taught our future doctors at medical school. As I begun my spiel, I felt really stupid. However as I continued, I saw her looking very intrigued at what I was saying, and nodding her head as if she was learning some of this stuff for the first time. "There's no way she doesn't already know this," I told myself. So instead of telling her stuff about nutrition, I started to ask her questions about nutrition – kind of like doing a quiz to see how much she actually knew. I started with the most difficult questions because I thought the other questions would be too simple. I was so shocked to hear her say, "I don't know." I was asking questions about nutrition to a top heart surgeon and I had the answers, but she didn't. It was incredible. But what was more incredible was that as I continued to ask her more and more questions, she had a very hard time coming up with answers, even the so-called easy ones. I was flabbergasted. (I love it when I get a chance to use that word!) So during my flabbergastinization, I guess I had such a surprised look on my face that she said to me, "Dante, I don't really know much about nutrition. In all my years of schooling to be a doctor, we were only required to take two nutrition classes, one in undergrad and one in medical school, and those were very basic nutrition classes. We doctors don't know a whole lot about nutrition, and that's why when patients need nutritional assistance we just refer them over to a registered dietitians. Why do you think I'm here with you?" And that was a super boost to Dante's confidence. I think I needed two pillows to fit my head on that night. I was twenty-one years old and I knew more about nutrition than one of the top heart surgeons in Southern California, and I was actually teaching her stuff. Moral of the story: doctors are not nutritionists. If doctors don't know much about nutrition, you can imagine how much the normal person doesn't know about nutrition. We eat multiple times a day, every day, for our whole lives, and hardly know anything about the basics of nutrition. So that's what this chapter is about. Again, there's so much conflicting information out there that it can all be so overwhelming and confusing. So the following is *all* you need to know.

Nutrition for beginners

In the first nutrition class I ever took at UCSD, I learned that there are only six things (nutrients) you need to ingest into your body (besides oxygen) in order to survive. Three of these things have calories and three of these things don't. (A calorie can be defined as a unit used to measure the energy released by food as it is digested by the human body.) The ones that don't have calories are water, vitamins, and minerals. But first, let's start with the ones that do have calories, I'm sure you've all heard about these: carbohydrates, proteins, and fats.

Carbohydrates

These are the body's main source of energy. They are the guys that make up all your starches and grains – bread, pasta, rice, chips, cereals, potatoes, and fruits. What happens to these in the body is that they are broken down into simple sugar molecules called glucose (blood sugar) that the body uses for energy. Our entire body – brain, nervous system, muscles, etc. – is fueled by glucose. Without energy we would eventually die because there would be no fuel for the body. So our body breaks down carbohydrates into glucose for immediate energy, and the rest is stored in the liver as reserves called glycogen. When the liver is too full, the excess amount is stored as fat.

Carbohydrates have 4 calories per gram.

Proteins

These are the building blocks of muscles and tissues. They are your meats, chicken, fish, turkey, egg whites, etc., as well as soy and tofu. Your body breaks down protein into amino acids for the growth, repair, and maintenance in the muscles and tissues of the body. Protein helps heal the body and maintain a strong immune system – production of blood cells, hormones, formation of antibodies, and building of enzymes. Protein is not a great source of energy, it is not used for fuel unless carbohydrate intake is limited, which can be taxing on the liver and kidneys.

Proteins have 4 calories per gram as well.

Fats

These are essential to health because they help deliver vitamins, minerals, and nutrients needed for normal growth and functioning of the body. They basically are all your oils and butters. They are broken down into fatty acids, and then are used for transportation, enzyme actions, as well as absorption for vitamins. Even though they have the same name, fat that you eat is not the same thing as the fat that is on your body.

Fats have 9 calories per gram. So as you can see, fat has more than double the amount of calories per gram than carbs and proteins. So it's not the fat that makes you fat, it's the calories from fat that make you fat.

Vitamins & minerals

I don't want to get into the details of what vitamins and minerals do in your body and bore you to death. But what you do need to know about vitamins and minerals is that your body needs them in order to survive, and they are essential for living a long, healthy life. Disease and sickness arrive when the body is deprived of certain vitamins and minerals. Most poor children in third world countries are not dying of starvation, they are dying of a lack of vitamins and minerals. This is what malnutrition is. Vitamins and minerals are the antioxidants that fight off diseases and cancers, and protect us. Mother Nature has put these valuable nutrients in the good quality food we eat. The fresher, the more natural, and the more raw food is, the richer it is going to be in vitamins and minerals. A lot of them are lost when the food is processed, genetically modified, fried, or cooked. So try to eat your fruits and vegetables raw and uncooked as much as possible; steaming them lightly is fine. I used to hate salads, but I forced myself to eat them because I knew they were good for me. One year, I did a dietary colon/bowel cleanse in which I was limited to only fruits, vegetables, smoothies, soaked almonds, olive oil, fiber, and lots of water for three days. At one point, when I was craving 'real food', my wife made a salad for me and put everything in it: spinach, mixed greens, kale, tomatoes, soaked almonds, onions, apple pieces, with olive oil and squeezed lime juice as the dressing. I'm telling you that this was the best tasting salad I had ever had in my life. For the first time, I could actually taste the salad and everything that was in it. Now because of non-organic farming and pesticides, the soil where fruits and vegetables are grown is not as nutrient-rich as Mother Nature intended it to be. Because of that, I would advise everyone to supplement themselves to get an extra boost of vitamins and minerals. The best thing you can do is to take any sort of green superfood powder everyday. (We'll talk about this more in the Detox chapter.)

I love water!

My friend Paula Abdul, who was a dancer her whole life, once said to me, "Dante, you drink more water than anybody I've ever seen in my life." I took that as a huge compliment. I could write a whole book on water. I might be the only person who would ever read it, but I definitely could. Isn't it odd that our body and the Earth are both comprised of about 70% water? Doesn't it tell us it's pretty important? We need water, we would die without water. We could go weeks without food and still stay alive, but we could only survive a few days without water. Water is responsible for almost every biological function in our body. It is more important than anything else we could put in our body. And do we get enough of it? Heck no! As I mentioned before, most of us walk around in a constant state of dehydration. Imagine all of the cells of the body and tissues being deprived of water. How can they function properly and most effectively if they are not properly hydrated? How well does a fish do with very little water? Your cells are the same. Have a horse take you through the desert, keep him really dehydrated, and see how well he does for you. The same goes for your body. I will go as far as saying that 90% of all headaches are caused by dehydration. Most people get a headache and the first thing they do is pop an Advil or Tylenol. It's probably not even the pill that relieves the headache, but the water they take with it that hydrates the body.

When people take that water with the pain pill, it's probably the first true glass of water they have had all day. We assume that headaches just come over us randomly, but do we ever stop to think, "How much water have I had today?" or "Have I been drinking much water since yesterday?"

Now, here is the situation with coffee and alcohol. If you have one cup a coffee, did you know that in order to maintain your current hydration level, you need to drink three cups of water? See, caffeine is a diuretic. When you take it, it tells your body to get rid of water. It's one of the effects of caffeine, you can't get around it. So if you are going to consume things that have caffeine, then you need to drink extra amounts of water, and prepare to pee! Same with alcohol, it will get rid of your body's water as well. Feeling bad with a hangover is mostly because the body is severely dehydrated. I remember my nutrition professor in college saying that if you were to drink a glass of water right after each alcoholic beverage you consumed (1 for 1), you would never get hangovers in the morning. Some people know a little about this and try and drink as much water after a night of drinking right before they go to bed. That helps a little, but it's too late. You would need to be drinking the water along with the alcohol earlier in the night, not just right before you go to bed.

Being hydrated will also keep you looking young. Do you know what's one of the main differences between a wrinkly old person and a young person? The older person is severely more dehydrated while the young person is more plump with water. The old person's organs, tissues, and cells are dried out from years of lack of water. We can all change that now by drinking more water immediately, and keep doing it consistently.

The pee test

"But how do I know if I'm properly hydrated or not?" People have asked me this question over and over throughout the years. So here is the simple way to tell if you are dehydrated or not, and by how much. When you pee, look at the color. If it's clear, then you are properly hydrated. If there is any color, then you are dehydrated to the degree upon how much color is in the urine. If it's slightly yellow, you are slightly dehydrated. If it's yellow, you are dehydrated. If it's orange-ish, you are severely dehydrated. If it's red, well… then you better go see a doctor. The only exception is if you have taken multi-vitamins or any food supplement that has a lot of vitamins. They'll make your pee have a greenish or really bright yellow fluorescent color to it – kind of like the color of Gatorade. This is from the B-vitamins and is very normal. You'll be able to tell the difference.

Drink water so you don't retain water

If you don't want to drink too much water because you're afraid you'll retain water and look bloated, think again. Like the similar principle to fat, our body retains water because we give it a reason to. It retains water because it is not getting enough on a regular basis. If we give it enough water consistently throughout the day, then it has no reason to want to store it. Take a camel, an animal that's known to store a lot of water, and look at its environment and the conditions it's in. A camel doesn't get water for days, so its physiology has evolved to be able to store big amounts of water to be used during those hot desert days of trekking. If that camel had gotten water throughout the day, everyday, then it would have no reason to store water. The same goes with our body. If you feel like you have a tendency to retain water, simply drink more. In the beginning when you start drinking more water, your body will not be accustomed to it and you will be peeing a lot more often. This will subside after a while when your internal water balance gets adjusted and your body and cells learn to properly utilize the water for hydration. All in all remember that the body is 70% water and drinking a lot and peeing a lot is a really good thing because you are constantly flushing out harmful toxins.

People die of dehydration, not superhydration

"Is it bad to drink too much water?" This is another question people have always asked me. Let's do this, let's take all the deaths and complications related to dehydration, and compare them to those related to drinking too much water. Need I say more? In regular life – as well as in the health, fitness, sports, and medical industry – I have personally seen and heard of hundreds of people that have passed out from dehydration. And I have even seen people being put in an ambulance because they had to be hydrated intravenously, or it could have been fatal. I have never heard of anyone who had complications or was hospitalized for drinking too much water. I myself drink tons of water and I have never had any problems or complications because I was drinking too much water. It just doesn't happen. If the body has enough water, it will just pee the excess water out. That simple. I can guarantee you that you will never have any problems from drinking too much water. No doctor is ever going to tell you, "Ma'am, your problems are from you drinking too much water. You're too hydrated and you need to cut back." It's never going to happen.

Alcohol is like liquid fat

If I were to say that you all had to stop drinking alcohol in order to lose weight, I would probably lose most of you. I'm not here to tell you to stop drinking. I just want to inform you of how many calories are in the alcohol you drink, so you are aware. I once had a client who I was doing personal training sessions with, as well as running her nutrition program. She was doing wonderfully on her food intake and her workouts. However, when it came to reassessing her weight, body measurements, and body fat percentage, they were staying the same. I was puzzled and I couldn't figure out why. All my other clients were losing crazy amounts of weight and seeing fantastic results, while she was staying the same. She was getting frustrated and so was I, because it didn't make any sense. I know that no matter who you are, if you apply what I'm talking about, it will literally be *impossible* not to see results. So at one point, I asked her if she had done her cardio exercise the day before. I designed a program for each of my clients, suited for their lifestyle. Hers consisted of doing cardio a total of three to four times a week. She said that she did do her cardio, and I replied with, "Great, what kind?" She said, "Well… I went out last night and danced a lot." I thought to myself, "Okay… well, dancing is a form of good exercise." But something didn't sound right. And then it hit me. I asked her, "Did you drink any alcohol?" Then she said, "Well… yeah, my friends always think I'm so funny when I drink, so they always buy me drinks when we go out. But I danced a lot. I even was sweating, so it was totally like cardio." I smiled and said, "How many drinks do you think you drank?" She said, "Three or four." Which means at least four or five. So I calculated the amount of calories that were in her four drinks and got roughly 800 calories. And then, because I was a college student at the time, I knew what young drunk people do after drinking – and I'm not talking about sex. They eat late night crappy food. So I asked her if she ate anything after they went out dancing. She said, "Well… we did stop by some fast food place because I was starving from dancing so much. I didn't want to write it down in the food log I showed you because I was kind of embarrassed." She told me what she ate, I calculated again, and got about

900 calories for her fast food. (Which is, by the way, an average calorie amount for a moderate fast food meal.) So from the alcohol and the food, she consumed about 1,700 calories. Since she said she worked up a sweat dancing, let's minus about 200 calories from her 'club dancing'. That left her with an extra 1,500 calories that she wasn't telling me about. In order to attain the goals she wanted, she was only supposed to consume a total of 1,500 calories a day. So on the days that she was going out, she was consuming that normal 1,500 plus an additional 1,500 from the alcohol and the fast food. Then, I asked her how many times she went out with her friends, and she said at least twice a week. Here I had been stuck trying to figure out why she wasn't seeing any results. One pound of pure body fat (which is about the size of a big fist) is 3,500 calories. So if she was going out and doing this twice a week, she was almost gaining about a pound of pure fat a week. But since she had the rest of her food and exercise dialed in, she – thank God – was staying the same.

We all know that eating fast food on a regular basis – let alone late at night – is going to be subject to weight gain. She knew that, and that's why she didn't want to write that part down. But she didn't know how many actual calories were in that fast food (twice as much as she would have expected). But the main other aspect that I'm talking about here is that she never stopped to think about the calories that were in the alcohol. As you read earlier, carbs and protein have 4 calories per gram. Fats have 9. Alcohol has 7 calories per gram, which is almost as much as fat. So you see, alcohol is like liquid fat. Most people can drink a lot of it, and a lot of the time it leads to late night bingeing on bad food. Not to mention the kind of bad food you want to eat the next day when you have a hangover. And let's be honest, how many people feel like working out or being physically active the next day after drinking? I could go on and on, but I'm not here to preach to you about not drinking, I just want you to be aware. Calorie-wise, your basic drinks – glass of wine, beer, shot of alcohol – all have roughly speaking about 150 calories. Add the fruity mixers to your favorite cocktail on top of that, and it gets crazy. Piña Colada and Margarita, 600 calories. Mai Tai, 650 calories. Long Island Iced Tea, 700 calories. Ouch!! Your best bet is to stick with white wine (lower in calories than red) or a light beer, and limit your intake. If you must do hard alcohol, use limes, lemons, and water to mix with. Also drink a glass of water or soda water with lime after each drink you have. This will help you stay hydrated as well as keep you from drinking too much, but still look like you're partying. Cheers!

Eureka! I found the magic formula!

How many calories should you be having each time you eat every 3 hours? After years of experimenting on myself as well as hundreds of clients, after years of working like a mad scientist in a lab trying to figure out the magic calorie formula that would work for everyone... I finally found it!!!

Dream weight multiplied by 12 and divided by 5

The amount of calories you should eat depends on your desired weight, or dream weight. Not the weight you weigh now, but the weight you want to weigh. So take your dream weight, and multiply it by 12. This number is the maximum amount of calories you want to consume a *day*. Now divide that total by 5, and that's how many calories you should be having per *meal*.

Here's an example. If you're a woman and your dream weight is 120 pounds:

Take 120 x 12 = 1440 divided by 5 = 288.

1,440 is the maximum amount of calories you should eat a day. So every 3 hours you would want to eat around 288 calories.

Here's another example. You're a guy and your dream weight is 170 pounds:

Take 170 x 12 = 2,040 divided by 5 = 408

2,040 is the maximum amount of calories you should eat a day. So every 3 hours you would want to eat around 408 calories.

Like we talked about the last chapter, in the normal waking state eating every 3 hours ends up being approximately five small meals a day (e.g. 7am, 10am, 1pm, 4pm, and 7pm). But again, if you happen to wake up late and have to go to bed early, then it may only be four meals (e.g. 10am, 1pm, 4pm, 7pm). So don't worry so much about the number of meals and total calories for the whole day, just focus on eating your particular amount of calories per meal every 3 hours. If it seems small to you, remember that you want to be hungry in 3 hours. Don't go over the amount of calories you should have, but it's okay to go under. If your body doesn't feel like eating all of it, don't force it. However, *do* eat something every 3 hours, even if it's just an apple. This is how the body knows it doesn't need to store fat. And always remember you're not eating three hours before you got to bed. This is how you are going to speed up your metabolism, so that it burns fat in your sleep. It's really that simple.

Small meals equal a small stomach

I remember back when I was in college, a popular magazine was having this contest for the guy who had the best body. At the time, I remember wishing I could enter the contest, but I knew my body wasn't good enough to compete on that level. The winner was this guy named Rusty. I met him years later in Los Angeles working on a shoot together. We ended up working together regularly and when we went to lunch I always observed what he ate. I remember specifically one time he ordered country-style mashed potatoes and he said, "I love Southern cooking."

I remember being really confused. How could a guy who had such a great body be so nonchalant about what he was eating? However, on a job years later, I finally asked him about how he ate. He told me straight out, "My stomach is like the size of a *pea*. I eat really small meals, but I eat often. I can't eat large meals because my stomach gets too full." He went on to say that he pretty much ate whatever he wanted, and didn't make a big deal about it, but the meals were super small. Naturally, without even really thinking about it, Rusty was doing exactly what this chapter is talking about – eating small meals every 3 hours, so the body can look its best.

Nutrition labels

When I was a teacher's assistant for my nutrition professor in college, I was amazed at how much biology students didn't know the basics of reading nutrition labels. If biology students didn't know, then who did? I think this is one of the most overlooked and under-read aspects of general 'food knowledge'. There are basically two parts on nutrition labels:

- The ingredients (I will talk about it later in the book).

- The nutrition facts box with the amount of calories, the serving size, the servings per container, the amount of fat, carbohydrates, protein, etc. Let's focus on what's in this rectangular box.

Nutrition Facts

Serving Size 2 crackers (14 g)
Servings Per Container About 21

Amount Per Serving

Calories 60   Calories from Fat 15

	% Daily Value*
Total Fat 1.5g	**2%**
Saturated Fat 0g	**0%**
Trans Fat 0g	
Cholesterol 0mg	**0%**
Sodium 70mg	**3%**
Total Carbohydrate 10g	**3%**
Dietary Fiber Less than 1g	**3%**
Sugars 0g	
Protein 2g	

Vitamin A 0%	•	Vitamin C 0%
Calcium 0%	•	Iron 2%

* Percent Daily Values are based on a 2,000 calorie diet. Your daily values may be higher or lower depending on your calorie needs:

	Calories:	2,000	2,500
Total Fat	Less than	65g	80g
Sat Fat	Less than	20g	25g
Cholesterol	Less than	300mg	300mg
Sodium	Less than	2400mg	2400mg
Total Carbohydrate		300g	375g
Dietary Fiber		25g	30g

Calories: Use this number to make sure that you don't exceed the amount of calories you are supposed to have to be at your dream weight.

Serving size: The serving size is the amount of food that equals the calories given on the label. You're going to have to watch out for this because here's where food companies can fool you. Let's take a small bag of chips that says 140 calories. So you think that the bag of chips you eat with your sandwich is only 140 calories. Think again. If you look closely, you will see that the serving size is 1 ounce, and unless you look on the front of the bag and see that there is 2 ounces, you will never know that you are actually eating a total of 280 calories from that little bag. This makes a huge difference when you're trying to eat meals that are 300 calories or less. And guess who's not going to be hungry in 3 hours?

Servings per container: Servings per container is the number of servings found in the entire container of food. A big bag of blue corn tortilla chips (which I have all the time and are one of the healthiest chips you can eat) says it has 140 calories. Now if you look at the servings per container it says 16. In other words, in one bag you have 140 calories times 16. So the whole bag of these healthy chips contains 2,240 calories. If you're one of those people who sit in front of the TV and can eat a whole bag of chips, you're consuming a day worth of calories in one meal. Remember that's how sumo wrestlers eat. Another example is in drinks. I like those Vitamin Waters. They have vitamins and electrolytes to help keep you hydrated and they don't have any artificial flavors or colors, which is really what I love about them. But if you look at the nutrition facts on these tasty drinks, you'll see that it says they have 50 calories. So you may think, "Oh that's not bad... I'm only drinking 50 calories." But if you look closely at the servings per container, you will see that there are 2.5 servings, which equals 125 total calories, not 50. So you see, it's important to always look at the servings per container when calculating your calories.

Now that you know how to read nutrition labels, you will have a better understanding of the relationship between calories, the serving size, and the servings per container. In the beginning, you are going to have to pay attention to these labels on the foods you normally eat, but don't worry because you will soon become familiar with everything and know exactly how much you should be eating.

Balanced meals

Earlier in this chapter, you read about the basic functions of carbohydrates, protein, and fat. So when you look at food labels, it is good to eat foods that are balanced in these three. For example, if you only have carbs (e.g. pasta) for a meal, your blood sugar levels are going to spike and the extra sugar from the carbs will have a tendency to be stored as fat. But if you have protein (e.g. chicken) with your carbs, it will help to stabilize your blood sugar levels and your body won't need to store the excess sugar as fat. There is a lot of info out there that may argue not to food-combine (i.e. eat your carbohydrates separate from your protein). If this is something that works well with you, and you feel good about it, then keep doing it. However, if you are reading this, chances are that you are not 100% satisfied with how your body is looking and feeling. Through my experimentations, I have found that balanced meals (ones that contain a mix of carbohydrates, protein, and fat) are best. Look at the basic food that we came into this world having, breast milk – a mix of carbohydrates, protein and fat.

The cheat day

Do you know where the expression *monster's ball* comes from? It's when they are about to execute a person on death row, and the day before, they let them eat whatever they want. If they want a super-sized #4 Big Mac at McDonalds with a chocolate caramel sundae with peanuts and a cherry on top, then they get it. It's a going-away present that the state gives the criminals before they send them off to heaven via the electric chair – so nice of them. Hence they give the monster a ball. So here's my suggestion to you. Even though you are not a monster – and hopefully not a criminal – give yourself a ball once a week. This my friend, is your cheat day. On this day, you can do and eat whatever you want. If you want to have cake and ice cream at that birthday party, then go ahead. If you want to go out for pizza and beers, then go ahead. If you want to eat like a sumo that day, then put your sumo diapers on because you are more than welcome to. Anything goes on your cheat day, and I'm suggesting that you honor it.

Now what is the point of the cheat day? Well, there are many reasons to have a cheat day, and most of them are psychological. Since this new way of eating is going to be a lifestyle change (and not a temporary diet) you want to feel free. Nothing is worse than feeling you are not allowed to eat something, having to always restrict yourself and be chained up in prison like that monster. This cheat day is your free ticket to have whatever you want once a week. And what I have found with others and myself is that you actually don't cheat all that bad. You'll be surprised. Sure, you may have some cake and ice cream, but you won't really want to eat the entire cake and the whole carton of ice cream. You may have a couple pieces of pizza and a few beers, but you won't want to eat the entire pizza and drink the whole 6-pack. You certainly can if you want, but you'll see that you now get full easily because your stomach has shrunk due to the other six days of the week eating small meals every 3 hours. When you eat a lot now, you'll feel way more full than before. There will be a huge difference between how you feel after a cheat meal and how you feel after your meals during the rest of the week. You'll see that feeling really full won't feel really good. Plus, you won't have much energy and will feel lazy afterwards because your body needs to go into a food coma to use all of its energy for digestion. (Think of how you feel after a Thanksgiving meal.) So even though you'll be enjoying your cheat day, you'll find that you now have a whole new orientation to food. You'll also have a new outlook on your body, and you won't feel like messing with it that much, especially after seeing the results that you will be seeing with actually not that much effort. Most of all, being allowed to cheat makes you not have such a strong desire to do so. But again, I really encourage you to honor the fact that you have a cheat day, and cheat as little or as much as you like.

A FEW TIPS

Don't eat out of the bag – Always pour chips, crackers, etc. onto a plate so that you can see the amount you are eating. Like I mentioned before, the worst thing you can do is to sit in front of the TV with a seemingly bottomless bag of chips. You can't tell how much you are eating when you are shoveling handfuls from a bag or box, not to mention being distracted while watching your favorite TV-show or movie. So just take out the amount you should be eating within your calorie range, seal up the bag or box, and put it back into the cupboard before you start eating.

Eat slowly – It takes about 20 minutes for your stomach to feel full. The digestion process starts the minute food enters the mouth, but it takes a moment for the food to accumulate in the stomach. The stomach will then stretch out and send a signal to the brain to give you that full feeling. So when you eat fast, you may not have that full feeling yet, and you may just keep eating. Whereas if you eat slower, you will feel satisfied at the right time. So really enjoy your food, and eat slowly.

Use a cooking spray – If you can, for the most part, use a cooking spray in the pan instead of oil. A lot of oils are good for you to cook with (like coconut oil), but oils do contain a lot of calories. A cooking spray contains none. So using a cooking spray will take a lot of calories out of your meals.

Eat the egg whites instead of the whole egg – A typical large egg has about 80 calories – not to mention up to 250 mg of cholesterol. Of the 80 calories about 60 of them come from the yolk, which means that only 20 calories come from the egg whites. So when preparing eggs in the morning, siphon out the yolk, and just put the egg whites in the pan – as best and clumsily as possible. For baking recipes, you can substitute two egg whites for one egg. You can now find cartons that just have egg whites in them at most grocery stores. And when ordering breakfast in the restaurant, you can ask for egg whites only.

Schedule conflicts – If you're on the schedule of eating 300 calories every 3 hours (you'd be burning 100 calories every hour), and it's time to eat but you have dinner scheduled in an hour, then just eat 100 calories (an apple or a banana). The main thing is not going four hours without eating.

Restaurant ordering – Let's be honest, when you go to a restaurant, all they care about is trying to give you the best tasting meal so that you will come back. The last thing they are concerned about in the kitchen is for you to have a low calorie meal. So this is your responsibility when ordering. Remember, you don't see them cooking back there. I know at first you may think you are being difficult when ordering, but who is paying for the meal? You are! So you can get whatever you want. If you are with friends and you think they may be judging you, think again. Like I said before, you will probably inspire them, and your physical results will speak for themselves.

No oil or light oil – I've been to some restaurants for breakfast and asked them if I could get egg whites, and when they bring the plate the egg whites are drenched with oil. So just tell them no oil or light oil, otherwise they might go to town. Remember, oil has a lot of fat, and fat has 9 calories per gram. And like you learned earlier, it's not the fat that makes you fat, it's the calories in the fat that make you fat.

Dressing on the side – You might think you are being healthy by ordering a salad for lunch, but do you ever consider the amount of calories that are in the dressing? One tablespoon of olive oil is 120 calories. One tablespoon of ranch dressing is about 75 calories. And how many tablespoons do you think they put in your salad? The packet of 1,000 Island dressing that McDonalds gives you to put on their salad is 390 calories! Yep... look it up yourself. So the best bet is to always ask for dressing on the side, so you can see exactly how much is going on your salad. Pure balsamic is a good choice. Also try using lime or lemon to flavor your salads.

Fast food – Most all fast food and chain restaurants are now required to list the amount of calories on their food menus. If not, all you have to do is ask for the nutrition information of their meals, and they will hand you a sheet with it on there. Plus, almost every dish at any fast food or chain restaurant is on the Internet with all the calorie and ingredient information. Check it out, you will be surprised.

Subway – If you're used to eating a footlong sandwich at Subway, only eat 6 inches now. Still order the footlong, but comfort yourself by knowing you're going to eat the other 6 inches in 3 hours.

Eat fruits and vegetables – Recently there have been a lot of rumors going around on how fruits are bad for you because they have a lot of sugar. First of all, to me, anything that grows from the Earth that is not poisonous and is edible is not bad for you. Processed sugar in man-made foods is not good for you, but the natural sugar Mother Nature puts in fruits is. The difference is that processed sugar – called sucrose – is very high on the glycemic index, which means it rapidly increases blood sugar levels, resulting in spiking insulin. The rush of insulin tells the body to start to store the excess sugar as fat. However, the natural sugar in fruits – called fructose – is low on the glycemic index compared to other sugars and does not have that heavy spike on insulin levels that lead to fat storage. In addition to having a lot of vital nutrients, fruits have a high amount of water and lots of fiber, which is good to cleanse the body and give you a feeling of fullness. When it comes to vegetables, they are so low in calories and high in cellulose (plant fiber), it can sometimes take the body more energy to digest them than the actual calories they contain.

In all my years of working with clients on nutrition and weight loss, I have never heard of anyone who was unable to lose weight or started gaining weight because of eating fruits and vegetables. It just doesn't happen.

THE RECAP

- Stay hydrated, drink enough water making sure your pee is always clear
- Drink three cups of water to every one cup of coffee to break even
- Limit your intake of alcohol, remember it's like liquid fat
- Calculate the amount of calories you should have every 3 hours:

  Dream weight x 12 ÷ 5 = ...
- Read the nutrition labels on the foods you eat to know the calories, and pay attention to the serving size
- Honor your cheat day as much or as little as you want

CHAPTER 3

EXERCISE OR EXTRA-SIZE

You may be one of those people that want to gag when you think about exercise. You may have made up your mind that there is no way in hell you're going to start a new exercise program. I have to tell you, if that is the choice you have already made, you will still lose weight in your sleep from doing everything else in this book. Now, that doesn't mean that I want you to skip this chapter, but it does mean that I want you to have an open mind. People have different lifestyles and comfort zones, so this chapter is for people from all walks of life to see what works for them.

Now I know what you're thinking, "I don't have time to exercise." Here's what I have to say about that. Exercise is about making a decision to do it, *no matter what*. I have known people who were the CEOs of multiple companies who still worked out everyday, and who also made time for their wife and kids. If you are one of those people who are saying, "But... I just don't have time to work out for two hours everyday," then you can relax because this is not what I'm going to be suggesting here.

Only work out 3.5 hours out of 168 hours in a week

In this chapter, I will be talking about doing a light exercise program where you work out every other day for no more than one hour. Not two hours. Just *one* hour, every other day. It's not necessary to work out everyday, I don't. We all have busy schedules, but there are 168 hours in a seven-day week. All I am suggesting is that you work out every other day for one hour, at the most. That equals 3.5 hours. 3.5 hours out of 168 total hours each week. I don't care if you're the president of the United States or someone even busier than that. I don't care if you have eight kids. Anyone can do it, even *you*.

What kind of 80-year-old will you be?

Everyone knows that from exercising you can lose weight and have a firm body. But did you know that if you exercise you will have a much longer life and it will keep you looking younger? In fact, from exercise alone, your body will function better, you'll have better posture and flexibility, stronger bones, ligaments, and tendons. And even more important, you'll have more energy and self-esteem. Now here is a question for you, do you want to live the last years of your life in a convalescent home, or do you want to increase your lifespan to be able to play with your great-grandchildren, enjoying life to its fullest, and being an inspiration for people around you? There are 80-year-olds who can barely move and need people to help them get around, but there are also 80-year-olds who run marathons. So it's up to you to decide today what kind of 80-year-old you want to be.

Toss the anti-depressant pills and grab a towel

Did you know that exercising increases your endorphin and serotonin levels? For those of you who don't know, they are responsible for you feeling happy and enthusiastic about life. This is exactly what anti-depressants *try* to do artificially, but what exercising will do naturally. Where do you think the expression *runner's high* comes from? It's not from potheads smoking a joint before their morning run; it's the euphoric feeling you get during and after exercise. This then contributes to an overall feeling of well-being in your life when you work out consistently. I've always noticed that I start feeling depressed when – for whatever reason – I haven't been able to exercise in over a week. That's why I always stay on my game when it comes to working out, so that I'm always high on life.

What does *tone up* mean?

There are only four things you can do to change your body: lose fat or gain fat, lose muscle or gain muscle. The expressions *get toned, thin up, more shapely, bulk up, put some mass on, lose some weight,* all refer to either one of those four or a combination of the two. For example, when you say that you want to tone up or get in shape, what you most likely mean is that you want to lose fat and gain muscle, which in essence gives the in shape and toned up look. If you have put on weight and have not been exercising, then you *only* have gained fat. You can't gain muscle if you have not been exercising – unless of course you've taken a new job as a construction worker lifting heavy equipment all day.

There's no such thing as spot reduction

Spot reduction is trying to lose body fat in only a specific place. Unless you're planning to get liposuction and have one of the most painful and longest recovery experiences of your life (oh, and by the way if you gain the weight back the fat is deposited in abnormal parts of the body), then you *can't* pick and choose where you specifically want the fat to be removed from. It will naturally be removed from where it's supposed to. Genetics do play a role here from person to person. Some people gain more weight in their face, others their hips, butt, or stomach. The main thing is not to worry about it, just do what's in this book and let Mother Nature take care of the rest.

The exercise program

In order to keep it very simple, I've broken down what your exercise routine should be into just two categories: weight training exercise and cardio exercise.

Weight training

The purpose of weight training is to build lean muscle. Why is building lean muscle so important to losing weight? First off, your body and skin will look and feel more firm, healthy, and contoured. Now, the other thing that's important to know is that muscle is a metabolically active tissue, which means that muscle needs and feeds on calories to stay alive, pumping and thriving just like your heart (which is a muscle). Fat tissue is a different story. Fat tissue pretty much just sits there and doesn't really burn any calories. It's just being stored. But on the other hand, muscle tissue is alive and active. So the more lean muscle you have, the even faster your metabolism will be. If you take two people who are the same height and weight, but one has more lean muscle tissue while the other has more body fat, the one with more lean muscle is going to burn a lot more calories during the night in his sleep.

Now, if you do the opposite and stop being as active or stop working out, you will lose muscle and slow your metabolism down. Why do you think people gain weight as they get older? It's not because they're just older, it's from not being as active as they used to be. So over the years, as their muscles have slowly atrophied (shrunk) and muscle tissue has been lost, the body has slowly gained fat because it has not been able to burn as many calories as it did before.

So do weight training in order to build lean muscle, look good, and speed up your metabolism. Let your muscles go to town and feast on your fat in your sleep.

Putting lean muscle on doesn't mean *bulking up*

People get confused thinking muscle is bulky and thick. But the truth is, all muscle is lean. People's confusion comes from seeing someone who started using weights and gained muscle, but they got really thick looking. This may even have happened to you. So now, you associate that look with using weights. But what actually happened is the body gained lean muscle but didn't lose any fat because of improper nutrition and lack of cardio exercise. And when you put lean muscle right under old fat, that's where that thick, bulky look comes from. If those guys and girls who lift a lot of weights and have that bulky look were to dial in their nutrition and get their cardio exercise on track, they would be lean and ripped. If you look at the anatomy of the human skeleton stripped of all fat, what is left is really thin, but strong and lean striated tissue. It's not thick, bulky, and puffy like fat tissue. Fat takes up much more space than muscle. So if you have five pounds of muscle next to five pounds of fat, the fat is going to take up way more surface area than the muscle. Imagine how much space a five-pound bar of steel would take up versus five pounds of marshmallows. Now imagine that same difference of muscle versus fat on your body. This means if you replace the fat on your thighs with the same weight in muscle, your thighs will be much smaller.

You won't look like a bodybuilder

When you see a real bodybuilder type who has an extremely low percentage of body fat and muscles on top of muscles, and muscles on top of those muscles, you have to understand that they have spent hours and hours at the gym for years and years with obsessive training and specific dieting, along with hundreds of supplements and enhancement drugs in order for their muscles to become that massive. It's abnormal and will not happen with normal weight training. This fact is important because I have worked with a lot of women in the past who feared using weights because they did not want to look like a bodybuilder. Right before I was going to train them with weights for the first time, they would always tell me, "Please don't make me look like those women bodybuilders." And I would always laugh and say, "That would be like me taking a golf lesson for the first time and telling my golf instructor, 'Please don't make me play like Tiger Woods'." It's just not going to happen. So the fear of ever looking like a bodybuilder does not pertain to you, I promise. Your goal is to put on lean muscle tissue to look toned and in great shape, so that you can see those natural curves and physique that Mother Nature intended for you to have.

Nothin' like the good ole fashion gym

I recommend that everyone should get a membership to a gym just to make your life easier. I know there are people who have a few old weights in the garage, some of which I'm sure have rust or cobwebs on them. You can definitely work out from home and I encourage you to stay consistent once you start. But for others, the home workout might get redundant and be taken for granted. The gym makes you have to really make an effort to get up and go, and you always come home feeling great with more energy. And since you are spending money for a membership, a lot of people feel guilty if they don't go because they would just be throwing away their money. Now, if you are one of those people who say you cannot afford a gym membership, I ask you this: can you afford to keep walking around with low confidence and low self-esteem? Can you afford to continue not to have any energy? Can you afford to be sick with a disease? Can you afford to keep having to go to the doctor and pharmacy to get that blood pressure and cholesterol medication for the rest of your life? Can you afford to have a heart attack or a stroke? Can you afford to not be able to play with your grandchildren? Can you afford to die sooner than you were supposed to because you didn't take care of your body when you had the chance? The average gym membership is about $30 a month. Are you going to let one dollar a day take control of your life and change your destiny?

If you still refuse to join a gym after my heart-wrenching pep talk, then it's okay. I know from experience that people will create any and every excuse not to work out, and will allow any and everything to come in the way of working out. And as long as in their mind they haven't made a decision to work out on a regular basis, they will always have something come up and get in the way. Just know that all you need to do is make up your mind that this is what you want to do, and this is what you are going to do, and everything else will fall into place. Eliminate any possible excuse. It doesn't matter what your situation is, you can still work out 3.5 hours out of the 168 hours in the week.

Get with the program

What should your exercise program consist of? Well, since you're only going to work out every other day for no more than one hour, I recommend that you work out each major muscle group once a week. So this would break down your basic weight training workout to what's called a 3-day split:

Day 1: biceps and triceps

Day 2: chest and back

Day 3: shoulders and legs

Since your abdominals are a muscle group that you can work out as often as you like, just work out your abs at the end of every workout.

I want to keep this as simple as possible. This is the workout I do, and this is the same workout my wife does. We both have the same muscle groups, so shouldn't we work them out the same? The only difference is that I'm going to be using heavier weights. If you refuse to join the gym because a dollar a day is going to break the bank, or the closest gym is two hours away and you would have to trek in two feet of snow to get there, or you don't have any weights or dumbbells at home and cannot afford to get any, then I'm going to show you a simple workout you can do at home with soup cans.

3-day soup can workout

Go into your cupboard and pull out two soup cans or any two cans that weigh the same. Remember, at the gym you can do the same workout, just substitute the soup cans for dumbbells. For each muscle group, I am going to give you two different exercises. At first, you only need to do one of them. Later, after your muscles adapt, you'll be doing both exercises. Also, in the beginning I recommend you do two sets of 12-15 repetitions, resting for about 30 seconds in between sets. And as soon as your body feels comfortable with the exercises, you can start doing the standard three sets.

Go to www.youtube.com/sleepandloseweight to see a video where I show you how to do the following exercises.

Day 1: Biceps & Triceps

<u>Biceps</u>

Bicep curls: 3 sets of 12-15 repetitions

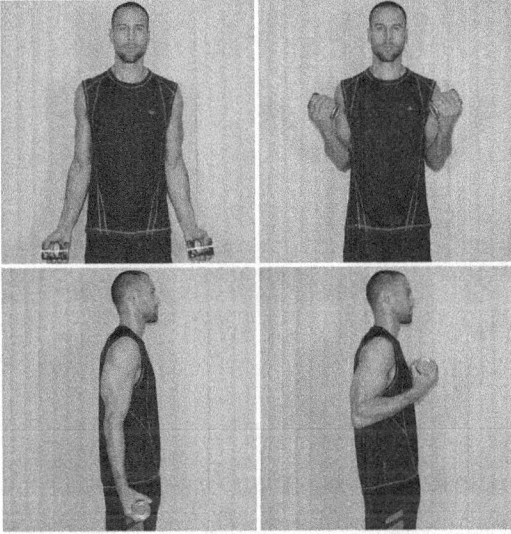

Hammer curls: 3 sets of 12-15 repetitions

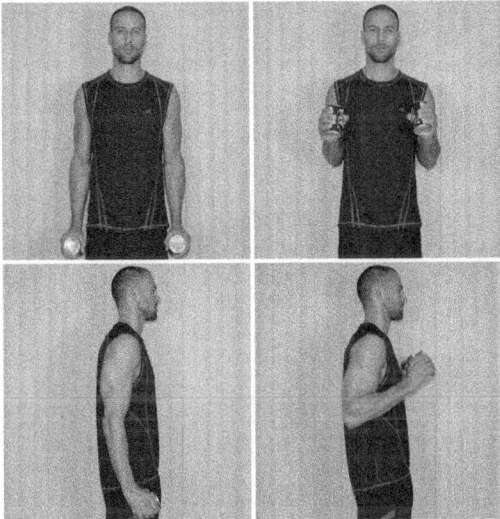

Triceps

Over-the-head tricep extensions: 3 sets of 12-15 repetitions

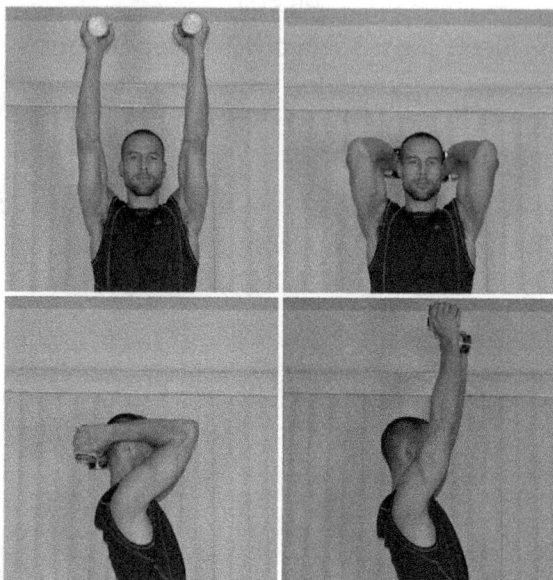

Tricep kickbacks: 3 sets of 12-15 repetitions

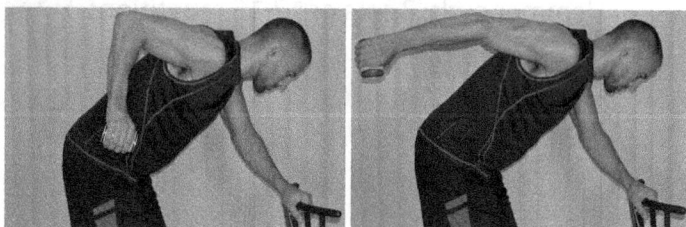

Day 2: Chest & Back

Chest

Chest press: 3 sets of 12-15 repetitions

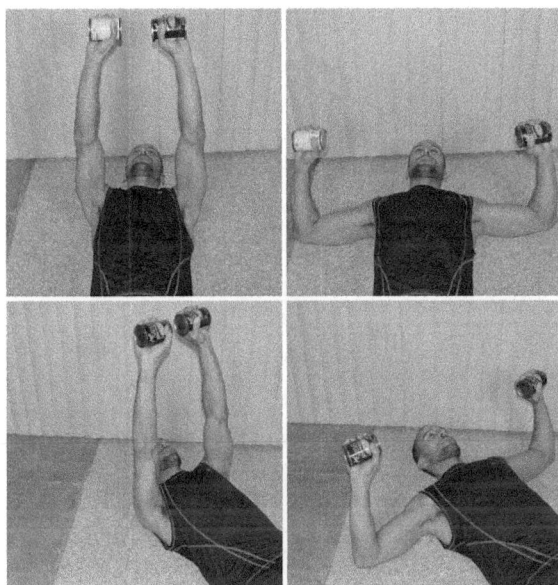

Chest fly: 3 sets of 12-15 repetitions

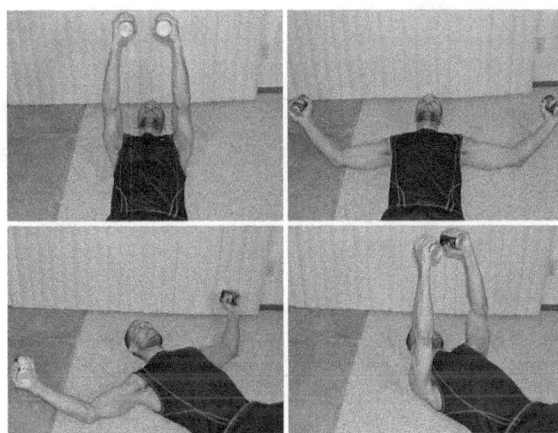

Back
Pull-over: 3 sets of 12-15 repetitions

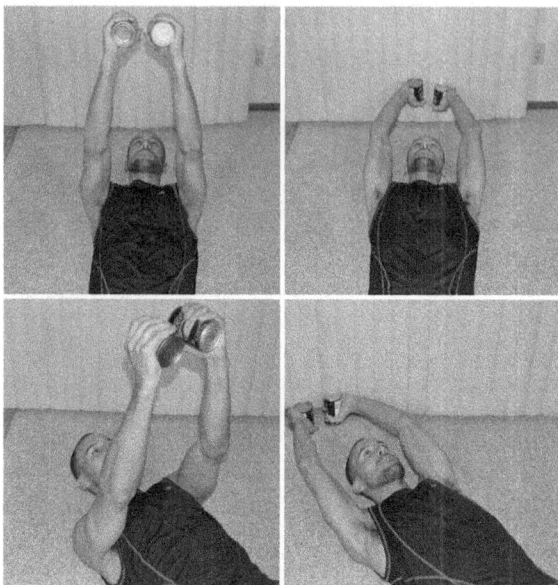

Row: 3 sets of 12-15 repetitions

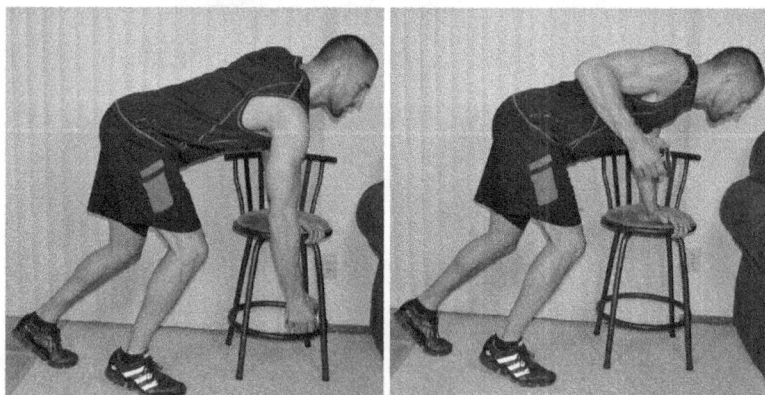

Day 3: Shoulders & Legs

Shoulders
Shoulder press: 3 sets of 12-15 repetitions

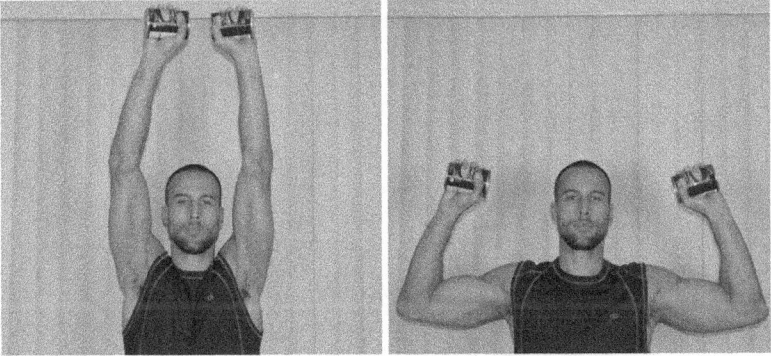

Lateral raises: 3 sets of 12-15 repetitions

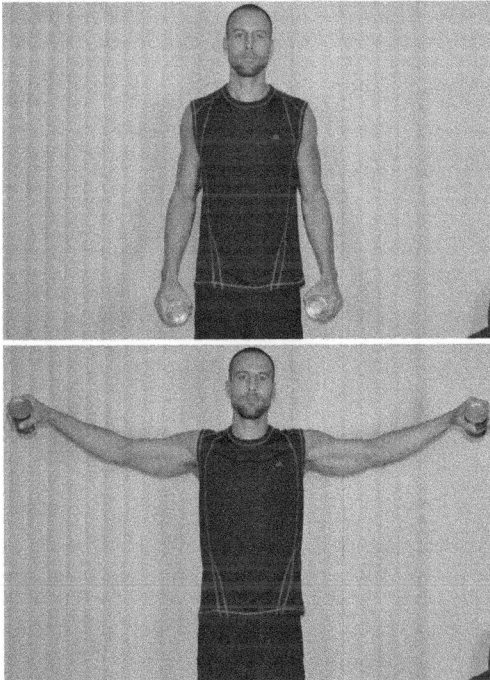

Legs

Body squat: 3 sets of 12-15 repetitions

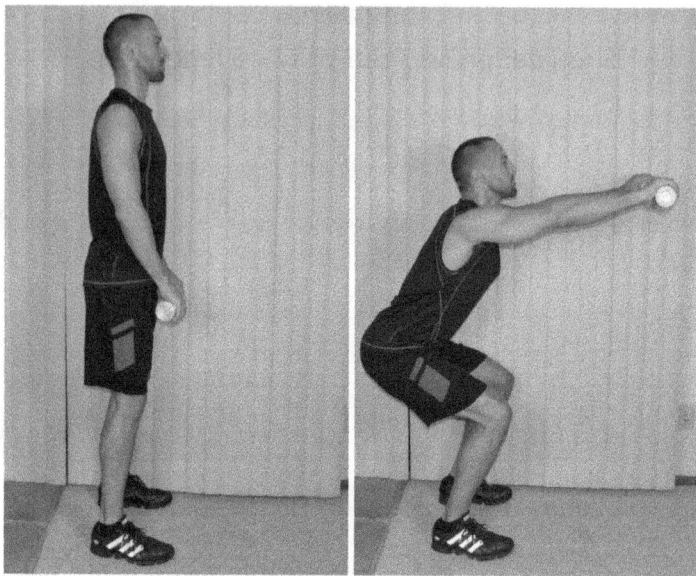

Lunges: 3 sets of 12-15 repetitions

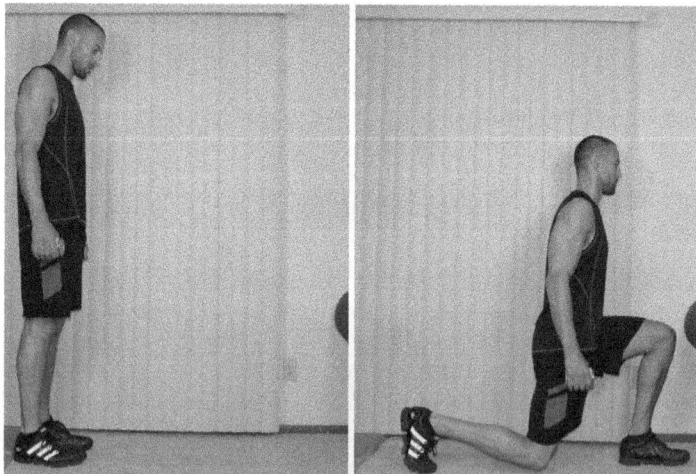

Calf raises: 3 sets of 30 repetitions

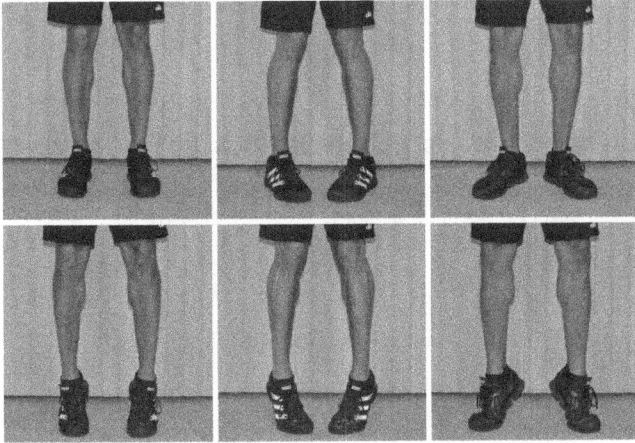

Abs

Crunch: 3 sets of 12 repetitions (or more if you feel comfortable)

Reverse crunch: 3 sets of 12 repetitions
(or more if you feel comfortable)

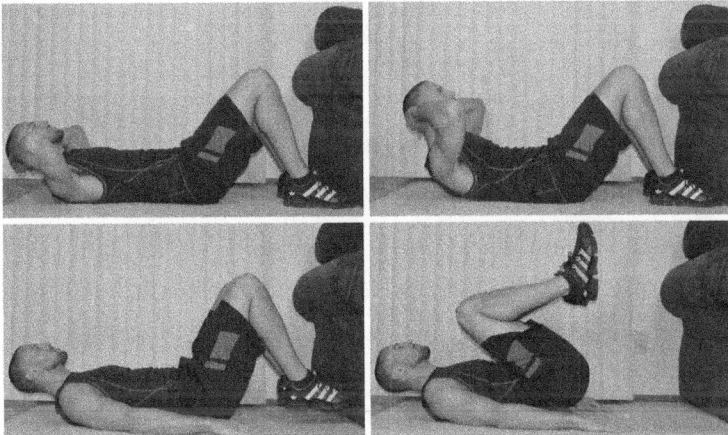

For those of you who don't have dumbbells and have never worked out with them before, soup cans are going to be a great starting point. But as soon as you get the hang of the exercises, the soup cans are going to be much too light. This will be a good time to go to your local sporting goods store and pick up some heavier dumbbells. Test them out before you buy them and see what weight works for you. Remember, if you want to see results and put on lean muscle to tone the body, you want the weights to be heavy enough to challenge yourself.

Cardio

Cardiovascular exercise is any sort of physical activities that are going to get your heart rate up for a prolonged period of time. These are your running, swimming, biking, spinning, rowing, stair-master, stair-climber, treadmill, dance cardio classes, step classes, zumba, etc.

There is a trick to cardio. This is something that has been so overlooked by so many people in the fitness industry trying to have a great body. They either don't know or don't pay attention to this. It is so important that I couldn't dare talk about or recommend a cardiovascular workout without letting you know about this key factor. You have to have your heart rate up to a certain number of beats per minute to be in a specific zone where you burn *body fat* for energy. If you're not, you will only be burning *calories*. Now, there's nothing wrong with just burning calories, because at the end of the day, calories that aren't burned will be stored as fat. But, if you're going to take the time to do cardio, don't you want to do it right? You may think this next section of simple math is annoying, but how annoying is it to be doing cardio for the rest of your life and never burn fat while doing it? I would never waste my valuable time doing cardio and having no idea if I was in my fat burning zone or not, and I don't think you should either. So here it is, the secret Karvonen formula[4].

The secret fat-burning equation

Wake up in the morning, and first thing before you get out of bed, you need to find your resting heart rate - how many times your heart beats in one minute. You want to get your true resting heart rate, which is with no caffeine and when you've been immobile for a while. Get a watch or clock, and with your middle and index fingers find the part on the side of your neck where you can feel your pulse. Count the beats for one minute. This is your Resting Heart Rate (RHR).

Now the particular zone you want to be in for your body to burn its own fat for energy while you are doing cardio is between 60%-70% of your maximum heart rate. To find this range, you're going to apply the Karvonen formula:

---

4 National Strength and Conditioning Association, *Essentials of Strength Training and Conditioning*, July 2000.

Take 220 minus your age

Subtract your RHR

Multiply by .60 (60%)

Add back your RHR

Tadaaa! The number you get is the minimum heart rate you want to reach when you're doing cardio.

For example if you're 30 years old and you have a resting heart rate of 70:

220 - 30 = 190, then 190 - 70 = 120, then 120 x .60 = 72, then 72 + 70 = 142

So 142 beats per minute is the minimum range (60%) you would want to be at. The same should be done for the upper range, just multiply by .70 (70%). The number you'll get is the maximum heart rate you should reach while doing cardio.

So now you know the range you have to be at when you're sweating your butt off... literally! It's that simple, and once you know this, you will always know if you are burning fat or not. I can't tell you how many people I have seen over the years pedaling nonchalantly on the exercise bike at the gym, casually reading a magazine or talking on the phone. They may be burning a few calories, but they are not burning any fat. Just so you know, the telltale sign when you are in your fat burning zone is that it is difficult to maintain a conversation. You can, but it definitely should be a struggle to do so. So just have your music on and do your thing for up to 30 minutes.

I want to add that a lot of cardio machines have a diagram graph of fat burning zone percentages lined up with age, so it can tell you how many beats per minute you need to be at to be burning fat. Unfortunately, these are incorrect. They take into consideration a person's age, but not their resting heart rate. So by their chart, they can have two women of the same age, one with a resting heart rate of 55 and the other one at 75, and it will give you the same heart rate zone, which obviously will be completely inaccurate. So don't go by these charts on the machines, go by the Karvonen formula that I'm presenting here.

Measuring your heart rate while doing cardio

There are three ways to know your heart rate while doing cardio.

First method: Use the heart rate monitor on your cardio machine at the gym. Just grab the silver handles, and hold your hands steady until the monitor reads your heart rate. From my experience, these don't work that well all the time. Sometimes they give a completely false reading or they just don't work at all.

Second method: In the middle of doing cardio, test your heart rate just like you did in the morning with your middle and index fingers on your neck. Just look at the seconds on the timer of the machine you are using. If you don't want to count your heart beats for the whole minute, you can just count for 30 seconds and multiply by two.

Third method: The easiest and the most accurate way to measure your heart rate is by using a Polar Heart Rate Monitor. (You can get them at your local sporting goods store or online for about $60.) These consist of just putting the polar heart rate strap around the bottom of your chest and wearing the polar heart rate watch, which picks up your heart rate. I have one myself and had my clients get these, and they were really satisfied. It's definitely worth the purchase.

Now, if you refuse to do this whole heart rate thing, I understand. Don't beat yourself up because it's too much of a stretch to count your heartbeat for one minute and do some simple math on your phone calculator. Even though you won't know accurately if you are burning fat while doing cardio, you will still be burning calories, getting your heart rate up, speeding up your metabolism, and getting major health benefits.

30 minutes is the new quickie

My workout recommendation is working your way up to doing 30 minutes of weight training and 30 minutes of cardio. Don't start out trying to do this much in the beginning if you haven't been exercising or if you have never really exercised at all in your life. You will build up to it. I remember the first day training my wife, she couldn't even do five minutes of cardio. But now, she looks back and laughs at that, easily doing her 30 minutes of cardio every other day. So take it slowly even if you only do five minutes or less of cardio in the beginning. Gradually start to increase, and you will find that it will become easier each time. It's perfectly fine increasing by only one minute each time you do cardio every other day. Soon, you'll be enjoying the results of doing cardio for 30 minutes.

Keep shocking your body

It's really important to mix up the machines that you do cardio on, or the method of cardio that you do. You won't burn as much fat or calories if your body gets used to doing the same machine or cardio exercise. Mix it up, keep shocking your body, and keep it guessing. Never let your body adapt to any form of exercise. Keep changing it up. If you're at a gym doing a specific cardio machine, I recommend that you switch it up every two weeks or so and start doing a different machine. Do the machine that you hate the most, it just means that you will burn the most fat.

Don't forget to stretch

Stretching helps with blood flow, recovery, and strength of the muscles, tendons, ligaments, as well as good posture. Make sure you stretch in-between sets when doing your weight training exercises as well as after you do cardio. The best form of stretching is static stretching in which you focus on holding the stretch (not bouncing) for 20 seconds.

Yoga is not new age anymore

A type of exercise that has been around for thousands of years, and that has gotten more popular in the United States in the last decade is yoga. Yoga is an amazing form of workout that combines mind, body, and spirit. It's great for strengthening the muscles, flexibility, and balance. There are all different types of yoga, so I recommend you try different classes and see which one is best for you. Yoga can totally replace a weight training routine, and some of the power yogas and hot yogas can definitely replace your cardio routine.

No excuse for excuses

For those of you who have slight to severe health problems or injuries, and won't be doing any type of cardio machines, just do what you can – even if it means walking around the block with an intention to get your heart rate up.

One of my clients didn't join a gym, but by doing what I told him from all that's here in this book, he still lost 60 pounds of pure fat. For his cardio, I just had him begin to walk his dog faster with the intention of doing it for a workout, rather than just for the dog's pleasure to poop and pee. It worked, and he got his heart rate up more, and he slowly began to increase the distance of the walks as well as the intensity.

I have seen a blind man come into the gym and work out three times a week. And he had a young son that he dropped off at the gym's childcare before each workout. What's your excuse?

I've trained an 80-year-old woman who was recovering from heart surgery, and who also had severe osteoporosis. The doctor told her that joining a gym and exercising lightly would be the best thing she could do for her health. She started working out every other day and said she hadn't felt that good in fifty years. I had her start stretching as well, and she swore up and down to me that she grew two inches. What's your excuse?

I've had paraplegics come into the gym and work out regularly, wheelchair and all. For cardio, they used what's called an upper body ergometer, which most gyms have. It's basically like a bike for your upper body that you pedal with your arms. Anybody can use them.

If these guys have the heart and courage to workout, then so can you.

THE RECAP

- Work out 3.5 hours out of the 168 hours of the week
- Work out every other day
- Join a gym if you can
- Do 30 minutes of weights
- Use soup cans if you don't have dumbbells to work out at home
- Check out www.youtube.com/sleepandloseweight for workout instruction video
- Do 30 minutes of cardio or go for a walk to get your heart rate up
- Use the Karvonen formula to burn fat while doing cardio
    Take 220 minus your age
    Subtract your Resting Heart Rate
    Multiply by.60 (then .70)
    Add back your Resting Heart Rate
- Stretch in-between weight training sets and after cardio
- If you don't want to do weights and cardio, do yoga

CHAPTER 4

PSYCHOLOGY OF YOUR BODY

Our mind creates our reality. I have trained people in health and nutrition from all walks of life for well over fifteen years, and I can say that hands down, no matter what you do or how you do it, you will not and cannot achieve the results you want without having your mind right. After working so many years with people on a physical level, I got to work with people strictly on a non-physical, mental level when I got my Master's Degree in Spiritual Psychology at USM. One of the reasons I chose to finally write this book was because I felt I had come full circle, knowing and understanding how mind and body were related and tied together. The goal of this chapter is to help you identify any possible misunderstandings or irrational beliefs that may be subconsciously blocking you. We picked up most everything we learned in life at an early age. The people who raised us taught us things and told us things that weren't always rational. In their book *Loyalty to your Soul*, Ron and Mary Hulnick Ph.D said, "A particular quality you can develop to assist in your endeavors to overcome challenges and grow spiritually is the *willingness* to question basic assumptions about what's true, because much of what people have learned while growing up is either not true at all, partially true, or seriously distorted." So I want to help you see if there is anything irrational you may not be fully aware of on a subconscious level, and help you to bring it to a conscious level. Once these things are brought forward and identified, *they no longer have the power they once had on you*; and they simply go away. With these potential mental blocks removed, the physical results you want will be more easily attained.

"Eat all your food, there are starving kids in Africa!"

An example from my life was my parents always telling me as a little kid to eat all the food that was on my plate. I was actually forced to do it or I couldn't get up from the table. For a while into my adult life, I would always finish everything that was on my plate whenever and wherever I ate, even if it meant being extremely full. As an adult, I was subconsciously doing what my parents forced me to do, and I wasn't even aware of it even though it was totally irrational. I now know that overeating is completely irrational and that it only leads to fat storage. When faced with the extra food on my plate, I now ask myself, "Would you rather store the extra food on your plate or on your body?"

The irrational belief: I am fat

Years ago, I met a guy who approached me to help him lose weight and have a better body. He was 5'10" and was about 220 pounds. He said he had once been semi-fit, but that it was many years prior and he just couldn't seem to shed the weight he packed on. So I got him going on my nutrition and fitness program - eating smaller meals more often, working out with weights, and doing cardio every other day. He lost about two pounds a week. (By the way, unless you're severely over-weight, scientifically speaking you cannot lose more than two pounds of fat per week. This is contrary to what some weight loss programs or supplements may claim.) Within six months, he lost 50 pounds of pure fat, which got him from 220 pounds down to 170 pounds. He looked like a new person. Unfortu-nately, a few years went by and slowly but surely he put the weight back on. He asked me once again to work with him to get his weight back down. He had been under a lot of stress at work and just wasn't able to focus on his body. But this time, when I worked with him, I decided to take the time and see if there were some deeper issues that were coming into the picture. I started asking him questions about his family, what it was like for him growing up in his household, etc. He told me that his parents divorced when he was really young and that his mom got remarried to his stepfather who raised him, and whom he pretty much referred to as his dad. He told me that his stepfather was always overweight when he was growing up, and still was to this day. I felt we were getting

77

somewhere, so I began to ask more questions about his step-father like what kind of person he was, how he behaved, what kind of things he used to say to him, etc. I know from studying psychology that things parents do or say to us at a young age can stick with us for a lifetime - knowingly and unknowingly. When we are kids, we are like sponges, and a lot of stuff goes in and stays in - rational and irrational. It turned out that, when he was a boy, his stepfather used to say to him that he was going to be fat when he grew up. Now, before we get all mad at the stepdad saying, "How could he be so cruel," let's look at it from a different perspective. *People don't know what they do. People do their best based on what they know at the time. And if they don't know any better, then that's all they can do.* The stepfather was overweight, and he was just *projecting* his own self-image on the boy. We all have done it, most always unknowingly. Other people and our environment are nothing but a mirror of how we see and feel about ourselves. *Outside experience is a reflection of inner reality.* The stepfather was feel-ing fat and saw fatness in others, and therefore projected that on them. His own dad most likely did the same to him when he was a boy. So all he was doing was repeating what he knew, but I'm sure he was completely unaware of it. Once my client realized all of this, we worked on him not having judgment and blaming his stepfather, and instead forgiving *himself* for buying into a false belief based on what his stepfather had said. You know as we were kids, our parents and authoritative figures (even though they were much older than us) were still trying to figure out life. They didn't have it figured out then, and probably still don't know. But as kids, we really don't know that, and we believe what they say and tell us, even though it may be completely irrational. Our job today is not to be mad at them and judge them. Our job is to go through and dissect what was rational and what was irrational. As a kid, this guy bought into the irrational belief that his stepfather was right and believed it on a subconscious level, and since our minds are so powerful, he made it true. So he could get on a good fitness and nutrition program and lose weight, but on a subconscious level he would still see himself as being fat, and would eventually fall off and gain the weight back. After examining it himself, he saw that what his stepfather said to him had no basis, and that he was just projecting his own self-image on him. He forgave himself for buying into the irrational belief that he was going to be fat when he grew up, and ever since then he's been able to keep the weight off.

How you look now is the result of the thoughts you had six months ago

People create their own fatness. Being fat is not something permanent, it's something one keeps creating. Six months from now you can either create another fat body, or create a thin one. The way you look right now is the result of your thoughts and actions six months ago. Six months are going to go by whether you like it or not. So are you going to lose weight, stay the same, or gain weight? Because it's *right now* that you are creating what you are going to look like in the next six months. We are constantly creating ourselves, and that gives a lot of hope because it means we can change the way our body looks at anytime if we want to. So take control of your next six months right now.

Forgive yourself for judging yourself as fat

In the first chapter, I gave an example with twins. Let's use this example again here in regards to the mind. One twin has the subconscious belief that she is fat, and the other one doesn't. Even if they both start implementing everything that's in this book, the one twin who sees herself as fat will subconsciously create reasons or excuses not to continue to follow this new lifestyle. And even if she were to do everything right, her subconscious mind would still make her have a slower metabolism than her twin because she still sees herself as fat. Either way, the twin that holds on to the irrational belief that she is fat, will never be as thin as the other, even if they do the same exact things. This is how powerful the mind is. This concept is one of the biggest reasons as to why people struggle so much with diets, exercise programs, crash dieting, yo-yo diets, and losing weight for a while but then gaining it back. For any of various reasons, on a subconscious level, they see themselves as fat. And if you subconsciously see yourself as fat, you can try to lose weight, but there is *a conflicting dynamic* taking place within yourself. It would be like taking two steps forward, but then unknowingly taking two steps back, and then wondering why it is so hard to get to the place you want to go to. The

job of the subconscious mind is to make whatever it is pro-
gramed with come to reality, and it is so powerful that it will
do so regardless of what it is. This is why keeping the weight
off will always be a problem until you get to the root of how
you see yourself and why, and correct any irrational belief.
Understand that whatever and whoever you have allowed to
give you a negative self-image was false. *All you need to do is
forgive yourself for buying into any irrational belief.* (E.g. "I forgive myself for buying into the irrational belief that I am fat.")
And it's always good to follow up the forgiveness with the
new truth. (E.g. "The truth is that I've been blessed with a wonderful body and I have the power to create it however I want
it to be.") Once you do this honestly and compassionately,
all the obstacles and blocks will simply start to vanish. From
there, your mind and your body will get on the same page and
behave in a *rational* way. You'll be able to easily apply everything you read in this book and see incredible results that will
last for a lifetime. You will lose weight in your sleep, and your
body will shift and restart to be how it was meant to be: lean,
full of energy, and feeling amazing.

The rational belief: I am worthy

While getting my Masters in Spiritual Psychology, I had to do
a myriad of real client/counselor therapy sessions with other
students. In these circumstances, as I was hearing the most pri-
vate and personal issues from literally hundreds of students, I
had to use the principles and techniques that we were being

taught. What I observed as the basis of all human problems was some sort of underlying issue of *unworthiness*. I found that everyone – including myself – has or has had to some degree, the belief that they are unworthy. I'm not clear as to how or why these unworthiness beliefs came into our minds – parents, society, religion, who knows. The fact remains that they are there, and they are irrational. Whether these beliefs come from something we did, something we didn't do, or something that we are doing, our own personal guilt may be the cause of the unworthiness. *Forgive yourself and move on, because your new body awaits you.* This is imperative because the mind is so powerful that if you have deep feelings of unworthiness, you may believe that you are undeserving of having the body you desire – a lean, energized, and healthy body that you as well as others find attractive. If you don't feel worthy, you could unknowingly be *sabotaging yourself* from ever reaching that. This is why identifying these beliefs, understanding that they are irrational, and forgiving yourself for ever buying into them, is fundamental and imperative to having whatever it is you want. Because the truth is, *we are all deserving no matter what we have done or what was done to us.* I truly believe that one of the purposes for our human journey is to overcome this irrational belief that for some reason we think we are not worthy of things in this world. As Ron and Mary Hulnick put it in their book *Loyalty to Your Soul*, "It becomes clear that self-worth and a sense of value – commodities you have been striving so hard to earn because of an unconscious fear and guilt that you've done something wrong – are nothing but mental constructs that have no meaning. You are valuable simply because you are Divine. Worth and value are inherent and cannot, and need not, be earned. They are intrinsic to your being." Feeling that we are unworthy or undeserving would be the same as if a flower felt it was undeserving of the sun. The fact that the flower exists shows that it is deserving of the sun, otherwise it wouldn't be here. Likewise, because of the simple fact that you are alive proves that you are worthy and deserving of anything you want in life. So forgive yourself for ever believing otherwise.

Change your thoughts to change your life

Science, philosophy, and spirituality have all been slowly merging, and we are starting to see and agree on how powerful our mind is. From documentaries like *The Secret* and many other books on the law of attraction, man is becoming aware and realizing how powerful his thoughts are. Many entrepreneurs, artists, and other successful people have talked about and written books on how their thoughts turned into physical reality. They first had to have the thoughts of what they wanted and believe it could happen, before anything came into physical reality. So if you have thoughts of abundance, then you will most likely tend to attract money into your life. If you have thoughts of good health and vitality, then you will most likely have a lot of energy and feel great most of the time. But this also works the other way around. If you have thoughts of sickness, you're probably going to be sick a lot of the time. If you have thoughts of being broke, you're probably going to be broke most of the time. Once again this is how powerful the mind is. So by knowing this, you can change your thoughts today, and be at your dream weight tomorrow.

Visualization

Right before you go to bed, visualize what you want to look like, be like, and feel like for 30 seconds. Imagine this as if it has *already* happened. Right when you lay your head on the pillow, close your eyes and visualize yourself looking in the mirror, seeing yourself as you desire to be, and let a smile come over you. Visualize people at work complementing you. Visualize yourself meeting up with friends that you haven't seen in a while who cannot believe how amazing you look, and are inspired when you tell them how you did it. Visualize yourself getting in and out of your car easily and a lot faster as your new body is so much lighter. Imagine yourself going into the back of the closet and pulling out old clothes that you weren't sure if you would ever fit into again, and as you try them on, they are actually too big now. Imagine yourself going into the clothing store and shopping for new clothes because all the clothes you have are way too big. Imagine yourself actually wearing these new smaller clothes. Do this (seeing yourself as if you have already lost the weight) for about 30 seconds right before you go to bed. The goal is to have a feeling of well-being, excitement, and joy with a smile coming over you at the end of the 30 seconds. (Feel free to do it longer if you want to.) Do it every night, and you'll see how powerful the results will be.

If visualizing yourself at your dream weight is difficult, my suggestion to you is to look at before and after photos of people who have lost a lot of weight. Pay close attention to people whose before picture resembles your current body type. This will help to inspire you on the transformation you can make. A great source to see before and after photos is the website www.bodyforlife.com (click on Success Stories). Not only can you find some real before and after photos of people, but you can also read their personal story which will help to give you some reality of similar challenges that they faced. In addition, you'll see that these people used similar concepts that I talk about in this book. *The Body For Life* program was a big inspiration for my clients and I when it first started, and I adopted many aspects of the diet and exercise philosophy in my life that have influenced these same pages you're reading.

Get the invisible monkey off your back

I have found that having unresolved issues with other people is another huge reason that prevents people from being happy and achieving their desires. After my mom and dad got a divorce, I was raised by my mom and stepdad from the age of five to fourteen, and then my mom and stepdad split up. My stepdad and I didn't speak to each other for the next twelve years. Here was a person who was like a father to me, who helped raise me to become the man I was, and we were on bad terms. Now, I repressed any sort of feelings I had about this for twelve years. I convinced myself that it didn't affect me and let my ego take over and continue the game of not giving in - as if I was benefitting from that. Not until the day came, twelve years later, that I finally had the courage to put down my ego and call him. When I look back, I realize how powerful it was for me and how much energy I was unknowingly exhausting all those years. Making that decision and taking action to get back in contact with him and be on good terms helped me see how much this situation had been impacting my life in ways in which I never knew. It was like an invisible monkey off my back, and it released an energy that had been blocked all these years. By handling it, I started to be more confident and happy, and consequently my life significantly improved.

I think most of us probably have this person or situation that can be resolved. If we really choose to, we can handle it. We may not want to because of our ego, or our judgment on what the other person did (too bad to be forgiven), or we don't want to take responsibility for what we may have contributed to the whole issue, or maybe we are just being stubborn and want to continue to be *right* instead of *getting along*. And all that is okay. No one is going to force you to do anything you don't want to do. This section just points out how making a decision to take the higher road and resolve these types of emotional issues with other people may remove blocks that could be keeping you from losing weight. Your body could be holding onto weight on a physical level, because your mind is holding onto unresolved issues on a mental level. *By resolving the issue and letting it go, your body will do the same and let the weight go.*

I personally have seen this happen many times. I knew of a young overweight woman who had been raised ever since she was a baby by her foster mom. But one day, she was suddenly given up to another family as she was still a kid. Her whole life she had felt abandoned and unloved by the person she considered her mother. Finally, in her adult life, she made the decision to find her foster mom and reunite with her. She found out that her foster mom had not given her up, but that the government had stepped in, and placed her with another family against the will of her foster mother, who then was not allowed to see the girl. So that woman had grown up feeling that she was unworthy and undeserving, but after reuniting with her foster mom and resolving this issue, she dropped a large amount of weight and looked like a whole new person. It honestly was unbelievable how much of a physical transformation this woman made from all the weight she lost and how happy she looked. Resolve the unresolved issue, and let it go. Your body will do the same with weight, disease, or any other physical ailment. Speaking from experience, I know it is not easy and it is emotionally challenging to make the decision to call or email the person you may be thinking about right now. It does take a lot of courage and letting go of the ego to make that first effort to finally give in, and resolve the issue. There's never going to be the perfect time. So maybe the time is now. Right now you can go ahead and do it. You have my full support and encouragement, and I praise you on taking that first powerful step. You'll feel so relieved after having that huge weight lifted off your mind and consequently off your body. Call that person or email them now. It's time.

THE RECAP

- Look for any misunderstandings you might have about food or exercising
- Identify any irrational beliefs you may have about yourself
- Forgive yourself for buying into any misunderstandings or irrational beliefs
- Know what the real truth is: you are worthy and deserving of anything you want
- Decide now what you're going to look like in six months
- Visualize your dream body for 30 seconds before you sleep
- Take the higher road with the person you have an issue with and call or email them now

CHAPTER 5

GETTING THE TOXINS OUT FOR A FASTER METABOLISM

Do you ever wonder why we need to change the oil in our car about every six months? They're not just adding oil; they're taking the old oil out and putting new oil in. What would happen if you never got an oil change? Do you think your car would keep running well? We all know that we have to do preventive maintenance for our cars – oil changes, air filter changes, radiator flushes, fuel injection flushes, etc. But it hasn't yet caught on that we need to do the exact same thing for our bodies. We have to understand that the medical industry is a business, and it makes money when something happens to us, not by *preventing* something from happening to us. Think about all the heart attacks, strokes, cancers, kidney stones, gallstones, and other diseases that could be prevented if we were to do regular scheduled detoxes on our body. But this isn't a preventive medicine book, so the main thing I want to talk about here is how your body can be in a better position to lose weight in your sleep if you get the buildup of toxins out of your body. Let's take for example a swimming pool cleaner

– you know those things that go around in the pool with a motor and a hose attached to it, cleaning up everything in the pool. Think of it as your liver – the filter of your body. What if the pool cleaner was never cleaned out? After a while, how well would it operate? How effective would it be to continue to clean out the pool? When was the last time you did a liver cleanse? When was the last time you heard of anyone doing a liver cleanse? Get my point. If you start to regularly clean out your major organs (colon, liver/gallbladder, kidneys) with a short 3-5 day detox, your body will be able to perform at its absolute best.

How does cleansing affect your ability to lose weight?

As you know now, the main thing you have to do to enable your body to burn fat in your sleep is to speed up your metabolism so that it is lightening fast. So let me ask you something. Take two cars at a NASCAR race; one car's engine is clumped up with old oil, dirt, and impurities, and the other car's engine is freshly cleaned out. Which do you think will go faster? Which do you think will win the race? The same exact thing applies to your body.

Additional benefits

Most people don't know all the benefits of doing detoxes. Being toxin-free and cleansing your body will benefit how good your face and skin look and will keep you looking younger. Do you think your body will age faster or slower with a bunch of toxic chemicals being stored in there from the years and years of bad food, recreational drugs, pharmaceutical drugs, over-the-counter drugs, alcohol, cigarette smoke, air pollution, etc.? Not only will cleanses help you look younger, but they will help you feel better, be healthier, have more energy, live longer, and of course... speed up your metabolism so that you will lose even more weight in your sleep.

Kinds of cleanses

Now I know what you're thinking. What kind of cleanse should I do? What should I start with? How should I do it? Here are the answers. From all the research I've done, I've found that a colon/bowel cleanse is the very first thing you should do, and you need to do it once a year. The two other cleanses I recommend are for your liver/gallbladder and kidneys. You only need to do them once every three years. It is recommended for the body that you do them in that order. So you see, it's not too much that you have to do. You probably get two oil changes on your car every year. Let's focus on putting more attention on our bodies and not our cars. When you have a heart attack, get sick, or get a disease, who really cares about your car. Your body is the most important vehicle you'll ever own.

Colon cleanse

First off, I'm not talking about a colonic, which uses a tube to inject water in the butt. (I've done these before and they're not the most fun way to spend your Saturday afternoon.) Here I'm only talking about a colon dietary cleanse – meaning you only need to change the way you eat for a few days. So why should you start with the colon/bowel cleanse? The colon or bowel (same organ) is your body's waste removal. When your colon is not working efficiently, your fecal matter is stored and becomes dehydrated and compacted in your bowel. Eventually, this waste turns to sludge and can slowly poison you by being reabsorbed into your bloodstream. If you don't have a cleaned out and well functioning organ that removes waste optimally, then how are you going to get rid of the toxins that are already in your body, plus the toxins that come into your body on a regular basis? This is why it is important to first clean out this guy. Once again, if you have a stuffed up and constipated bowel, do you think your metabolism is going to be fast? Here's something that's gross. Famous actor John Wayne who died of stomach cancer had an autopsy that revealed his colon weighed 82 pounds at the time of death. 77 pounds were composed of dried fecal matter. Now that's gross! He was a great actor, but unfortunately his diet and colon weren't so great. You guys don't want to keep storing fat, but I'm sure you don't want to keep storing fecal matter either.

A recommendation for a colon cleanse is the one by Dr. Schulze ($60 on www.herbdoc.com). I have no ties with Dr. Schulze, I just happen to like his products. Back in the day, Dr. Schulze used to operate a successful naturopathic health clinic before the government shut it down. People who wanted an alternative treatment of their ailments and diseases went there. He stated that whoever walked into the clinic did two things before he began to treat them: stop smoking (he refused any person who refused to stop smoking) and do his 5-day bowel cleanse – along with taking green superfood powder. (I will talk about this later in the chapter.) He says, to his continued astonishment, that 90% of his clients never had to get treated any further because their ailments disappeared after doing the bowel cleanse. That's how powerful doing a colon cleanse is. Personally, I have bought this particular cleanse for every single person in my family. Growing up, my mom was always constipated. So when I bought the whole family one of these 5-day bowel detox programs, I got her to do it, and she was overwhelmed with the results. This was years ago, and to this day she tells me, "Dante I had been constipated my whole life, but I haven't been ever since I did that cleanse." Now she'll probably kill me because I told everyone. I also got my stepfather the same cleanse and afterwards I put him on the whole losing-weight-in-your-sleep program. He ended up losing 60 pounds. I knew that his body was in a much better position to lose weight faster and more efficiently after his bowel was cleaned out.

So on Dr. Schulze's 5-day bowel cleanse, you are simply taking two sets of pills: one set contains herbs to naturally get your colon working and the other set contains fiber to clean out the colon. While doing the detox, you want to stay away from any animal products (e.g. meat, eggs, dairy) because they take longer to be digested and they have no fiber – which is what you want to avoid as much as possible on a cleanse. Avoid alcohol, artificial foods, processed foods, chemicals, or preservatives. Try not to eat anything unnatural during the five days. Eat as many fruits and vegetables as you like and drink lots of extra water. By the way when you do this cleanse you will *not* be on the toilet all day like you're having Montezuma's Revenge. You may go an extra 1 or 2 times per day, but not anything crazy that you'll need to tell your boss to get time off for.

From not doing regular colon cleanses, I believe hundreds of thousands of people die each year because they have a poor functioning colon that is literally packed with old poisonous fecal matter that is being reabsorbed into their bloodstream causing all sorts of problems. And most are not even aware of it. So do a colon cleanse to feel great, be healthier, and have your body functioning at its best.

"The secret to creating powerful health is cleaning out your eliminating organs, and the best place to start is your bowel!"

- Dr. Schulze

Liver/gallbladder cleanse

Your liver is the largest organ inside your body and it is also one of the most important. Its main job is to filter the blood coming from the digestive tract before passing it to the rest of the body. Without your liver, you couldn't absorb nutrients or get rid of toxic substances. Now can you see how important it is to clean out this filter once in a while? Imagine never cleaning out the filter on your car, dryer, or vacuum cleaner. You can get a 5-day liver cleanse from Dr. Schulze that involves having his herbal tea and drops, and eating whole fruits, vegetables, and juices.

The gallbladder is a small pouch that sits just under the liver. It acts as a storage vessel of bile for the liver. Bile helps to break-down and digest fats. The liver and gallbladder are connected to each other, so when you're doing a liver/gallbladder cleanse you are cleaning out both of these. Have you ever heard of people who have had gallstones or surgery to remove their gallbladder? I believe this can all be prevented by doing a liver/gallbladder flush to remove the gallstones that are in the gallbladder and liver. A great book to do this kind of cleanse is called *The Liver and Gallbladder Miracle Cleanse* by Andreas Moritz. (If you don't want to read the whole book, the actual cleanse is in chapter 4.) It's a very simple 5-day cleanse where the only dietary restriction is no animal products. It involves drinking extra apple juice in order to soften the gallstones, and on the sixth day taking a combination of Epson salt water, grapefruit juice, and olive oil. This will make hundreds of gallstones come out the next day. You're supposed to do it a couple times in order to get all the gallstones out. It truly is an amazing cleanse. I guarantee you will be surprised with the results. I surely was!

I believe that doing liver/gallbladder cleanses every couple years can help to prevent complications of the liver, liver transplants, liver failure, etc. Again the medical industry won't tell you this, because they don't make any money in doing so.

"Most ALL health problems, including serious and life-threatening ones, develop months, even years, after your liver failed to keep your blood clean."

- Dr. Schulze

Kidney cleanse

The kidneys' job is to filter and remove undesirable substances from blood plasma. Everyday they process about 200 quarts of blood to sift out about two quarts of waste products and extra water. Aside from removing waste, the kidneys also keep the volume of water in your body constant, help regulate blood pressure, stimulate the making of red blood cells, and maintain your body's calcium levels. Overtime, if the kidneys are not taken care of, people end up getting painful kidney stones, need kidney dialysis, and/or kidney transplants. Again, I believe this can all be prevented by doing a simple kidney cleanse every few years. Once more, doctors won't tell you this. It's sad to say, but they are not taught or trained to do so, the system just isn't set up that way. Do you think the car repair industry would tell you things to prevent your car from ever breaking down or needing to be repaired? No, they would go out of business. Same goes with the medical industry. So you have to take your own preventive measures to avoid these health problems. I recommend Dr. Schulze's kidney cleanse or getting the *Kidney Flush Combo* endorsed by Andreas Moritz (available on www.rainforestnaturalpharmacy.com). Both entail using herbal drops and tea. Pretty simply to help prevent any future problems with your kidneys.

Do your own research

You can get cleanses from all different sources. At your local natural food store, you can get them in the supplement aisle. You can also get them from companies that you trust on the Internet. You can research and find anything you want online, and I advise you to do so. A lot of companies have ratings and reviews of products online that are very helpful. One website I really like that I am a member of ($9.95 a month) is www.natural-cures.com. They have great step-by-step detailed cleanses and detoxes (from very simple to more advanced), as well as other great information on natural health. It doesn't matter where you get your cleanses, what really matters is that you do them.

Keeping toxins out

After doing a cleanse, you want to keep flushing toxins out of your body. To do so, eat plenty of fruits, vegetables, and fiber daily. Get a cereal that's really high in fiber like *Raisin Bran*, *Kashi*, *Fiber One*, or anything else that has at least 5g of fiber per serving (look at the nutrition facts to see this).

Now in order to prevent the toxins from going in, avoid processed foods and keep it natural as much as possible. Look at the ingredients (below the nutrition facts box) in the food you're eating. *If you cannot pronounce it, it's probably not good for you.* The smaller the number of ingredients, the healthier the food is… period. Avoid when it says artificial flavors, artificial colors, monosodium glutamate (MSG), and preservatives. Here's something that's gross about preservatives. The owners of embalming businesses (the people who treat dead bodies) have started using less and less embalming chemicals to preserve the bodies because people now have so much preservatives in their bodies from all the food they eat. Sick right? Plus, if you eat foods with preservatives, how do you expect to lose weight when there is food being *preserved* in your body? Chemical preservatives allow the food to have an extended shelf life, so the food can last longer at the factory and in your cupboard. However, you don't want it to last longer in your body, do you? Gross! So try and stick with foods that are natural or organic. Food manufacturers are catching on by producing foods that are more natural. They are priding themselves on labeling their products as being natural with no artificial flavors or preservatives. That's great for them, and better for us!

Your deodorant stinks!

Here's the deal with deodorants. Aluminum and parabens are active ingredients used in antiperspirants/deodorants. According to the National Cancer Institute, "Aluminum-based compounds form a temporary plug within the sweat duct that stops the flow of sweat to the skin's surface. Some research suggests that aluminum-based compounds that are applied frequently and left on the skin near the breast, may be absorbed by the skin and cause estrogen-like (hormonal) effects. Because estrogen has the ability to promote the growth of breast cancer cells, some scientists have suggested that the aluminum-based compounds in antiperspirants may contribute to the development of breast cancer."[5] In a 2004 study, parabens (which are chemical preservatives) were found in 18 of 20 samples of tissue from human breast cancer.[6] Underarm shaving allows parabens and aluminum to be directly absorbed into the blood stream through razor nicks. These toxic substances are then deposited under the skin in the lymph nodes, adding to the build-up of toxins that can't be eliminated because of the clogged pores. The lymph nodes are part of the lymphatic system that consists of a network of vessels that make up the majority of our immune system, which fights disease and eliminates toxins. The lymphatic system affects every organ and cell in the body, and when it becomes blocked, the body cannot effectively eliminate toxic material. A lymphatic system overloaded with toxic waste is the ideal environment for the onset of numerous illnesses, including cancer. The chemicals in antiperspirant/deodorants

5 The National Cancer Institute, "Antiperspirants/Deodorants and Breast Cancer," *Fact sheet: Risk Factors and Possible Causes*, Jan 2008.

6 Darbre PD, Aljarrah A, Miller WR, et al, "Concentrations of parabens in human breast tumors," *Journal of Applied Toxicology*, 2004.

can clog up the lymph nodes, making it hard for the lymphatic system to perform its job, and causing a high concentration of toxins, which can possibly lead to cells mutating into cancer. In 2003, Dr. Kris McGrath studied breast cancer survivors, and found that women who used antiperspirant/deodorant and shaved their underarms more aggressively had a diagnosis of breast cancer twenty-two years earlier than the non-users.[7] Men have a lower risk of breast cancer because they do not shave their underarms and their underarm hair keeps chemicals in antiperspirants/deodorants from being absorbed by the pores of the skin.

The bottom line is that these antiperspirant/deodorants have chemical toxins in them that can clog up your body, and prevent other toxins from getting out. Toxin build-up prevents the body from being able to function optimally, and when the body can't function optimally either can the metabolism. And if your metabolism can't function optimally, then you won't be able to burn off unwanted fat optimally. So even if you think the whole deodorant-cancer thing is BS, then you may want to make a switch for the sake of losing weight. Now I'm not suggesting that you stop using deodorant and stop shaving, but I am asking you to be more conscious and aware of the type of product you are using and what's in it. You can look at the ingredients to see if your deodorant contains aluminum

7 Dr. Kris McGrath, "An earlier age of breast cancer diagnosis related to more frequent use of antiperspirants/deodorants and underarm shaving," *European Journal of Cancer Prevention*, Dec 2003.

or parabens. I have done my own personal research on using almost every type of natural aluminum/paraben-free deodorant and I can honestly say that, unfortunately, a lot of them suck! However, through all my trial and error, I have found the very best one of all and I will be using it until I die. It's made by a company called Alvera (*Aloe & Almonds* is the one I use). I buy it on www.vitacost.com (which by the way is an amazing website to get the lowest prices on natural products, cosmetics, supplements, nutrition bars etc.). I always get *Aloe & Almonds* by the dozen and give it away to my family and friends, and encourage as many people as I can to buy it. Too bad I don't own a stake in the little company that makes this deodorant. But if they ever go out of business, I will take those ingredients and make my own in a lab if I have to. There have been times in the past when I have run out of this product and reverted back to what I used to use, and there is no comparison. For me, it works better than the biggest brands, and the people I know who have used it all say the same. It smells really nice and it does a wonderful job keeping you dry. So it's a win-win situation with this product, and that's why I love it so much.

Sugar-free is not weight-free

I used to drink a lot of diet soda. I thought it was great, it had caffeine and best of all it had no calories. But I noticed that after I drank a whole bunch of it, for days after I would feel a little dizzy, disorientated at times, with blurred vision. Then I came across an article that related these effects to the aspartame that's in diet sodas.[8] So I looked into and heavily researched aspartame. What I found is that the chemical aspartame is very similar in chemical structure to a glucose molecule (simple sugar), and the brain assimilates it as if it were a sugar molecule. But it's not! So who really knows about the short-term side effects (not to mention the possible long-term effects) of having a lot of aspartame. But the main reason I am talking about artificial sweeteners here is that several large-scale research studies have shown that people who consumed artificial sweeteners gained more weight than those who didn't. It was also observed that people had increased hunger with aspartame water versus sugar water.[9] See, aspartame contains methanol. Methanol turns into formaldehyde when its temperature reaches 86 degrees. (For those of you who don't know, formaldehyde is the chemical preservative used to preserve dead frogs for dissection in science classes.) And what is our internal body temperature? 98.6 degrees. So upon ingestion, the artificial sweetener aspartame is converted to formaldehyde in our bodies. And guess where formaldehyde

---

8 H.J. Roberts, "Aspartame (NutraSweet) associated confusion and memory loss: A Possible Human Model For Early Alzheimer's Disease," *Abstract 306, Annual Meeting of the American Association for the Advancement of Science*, Boston, February 13, 1988.

9 Qing Yang, "Gain weight by 'going diet'? Artificial sweeteners and the neurobiology of sugar cravings," *Yale Journal of Biology and Medicine*, June 2010.

is stored? In the fat cells! (Particularly in the hips and thighs.)[10] So my dear diet-soda lovers, the fat on your hips and thighs is being preserved by your favorite artificially sweetened drink. So if you want to drop the fat, my advice is that you drop the diet soda. I would recommend giving up sodas all together or just having them on your cheat day. But if you are going to drink sodas, drink the regular stuff, not only for the health reasons, but also for the weight reasons. And if you're going to drink regular soda, just remember there's almost 150 calories in a can, so don't forget to work that into your total calories per meal.

Stevia: the choice of a new generation

A natural calorie-free sweetener that I use every day and highly recommend is stevia. It is derived from a leaf, so it's 100% natural, therefore has no unwanted side effects. Big food and drink manufacturers are getting smart and are starting to put stevia in their products instead of the other chemical artificial sweeteners. The reason why it has taken so long is because you can't put a patent on something like the stevia leaf because it grows naturally. However, they are now marketing their own stevia brands (*SweetLeaf*, *Truvia*, *Stevia in the Raw*, etc.), which is great because everyone wins. They get the money and we get our health. Actually, I advise the artificial sweetener manufacturers and the people who manufacture

---

10 P. Humphries, E. Pretorius, H. Naudé, "Direct and indirect cellular effects of aspartame on the brain," *European Journal of Clinical Nutrition*, April 2008

products that contain artificial sweeteners to stop consuming these products themselves, for health and weight reasons. And I also advise their families to do the same. And if they can, they should invest their money and interest in branding stevia products as they phase out the chemical artificial sweetener products. *Vitamin Water* is already doing it with their *Vitamin Water Zero* line that is sweetened with stevia and has no calories. I always have them in the fridge. I will praise the day when diet sodas switch from artificial sweeteners to stevia. That will be the day I know that food manufacturing in America is changing for the better.

Now what are your best choices for drinks when you are eating out? Obviously water is going to be your healthiest and best choice. Chilled water or water with ice is even better because the body has to warm it up when it's going down. Drinking eight ounces of cold water can burn off an additional 9.25 calories compared to room-temperature water. I did the math and by drinking the recommended 8 cups of water per day, if it is ice cold we would end up burning about 8 pounds of pure fat a year. Those who don't like the taste of water may want to try flavoring it with sliced cucumbers, lemon, stevia, etc. The second best choice would be an unsweetened iced tea. Again, you can squeeze lemon in it and sweeten it up with stevia if you want. Stevia isn't widely offered at restaurants yet, but you can buy packets at your local health food store and many conventional grocery stores are now beginning to carry it. So if you buy a box of these packets you can always have a few with you in your bag or purse. I always keep a few in the glove compartment of my car. If you are against having stevia, then I next recommend agave nectar or honey. If none of those are available, I next recommend *Sugar in the Raw*. These are the brown packets that are natural unprocessed sugar. This type of sugar is way better for you than bleached white sugar. However, I still would recommend white sugar over the blue packets (aspartame), over the pink packets (saccharine), and even over the yellow packets (sucralose, toxic chlorinated glucose).

Pipe down on the prescriptions if you can

My last recommendation to keep the toxins out to enable your body to optimally burn fat in your sleep is to look to slowly lower or wean yourself off prescription medications if you don't really need them. Doctors are good people who are taught to prescribe medication. But you are in charge. If you really don't think you should be taking a medication or if you feel it's time to get off a medication, then take the initiative and tell your doctor. Deep down we truly know what's best for us, and if you feel that you are taking a drug that's unnecessary, then speak up. Medications are chemicals which are all toxic to some degree in our bodies and are very taxing on the liver and kidneys that have to work overtime to filter them out. So why not take some pressure off your organs so that they can do other jobs? Obviously, in a lot of cases, people need their medications for serious health issues, and luckily we have a medical association that can aid in these severe problems. But I'm mainly talking about medications that some of us really don't need to be taking or for those who feel that maybe it's time for them to come off a particular medication. So if you feel it's time, ask your doctor if you can slowly come off a medication. If you are taking any type of beta-blockers, blood pressure medication, or any cholesterol medication, you'll see that your blood pressure and cholesterol levels will significantly lower when you start implementing what's in this book. This new lifestyle will directly lower these ailments, so that you may not need to take those medications anymore. I have watched my clients time and time again lower their blood pressure and cholesterol levels to impressive measures to which even I was shocked.

The wonderful green superfood powder!

The one supplement I highly recommend for overall health, vitality, energy, nutrients, and daily detox is green superfood powder. It's a highly concentrated form of super nutrition to fortify your body. Most superfood green powders contain some sort of blend of wheat grass, barley grass, alfalfa grass, chlorella, spirulina, kelp, kale, broccoli, spinach, and parsley. These powerful green foods are some of the most nutrient dense whole foods grown on Earth that provide the richest form of vitamins and minerals to feed, cleanse, repair, and energize your body on a cellular level. Dr. Schulze has a really good superfood powder that you can order along with his cleanses. (When I bought everyone in my family his bowel cleanse, I also bought them his superfood to go along with it.) But the green superfood powder doesn't have to come from Dr. Schulze. There are dozens of brands out there that you can get online or in the health food section of most grocery stores. Natural food stores will have an even bigger variety. Trader Joe's has an excellent one that's cheap called *Super Green Drink Powder*. I've tried them all and liked them all, so choose your favorite one. I personally have at least 1-2 scoops everyday. First thing in the morning, I go down and put a scoop of green superfood in 2-4 ounces of natural apple juice, shake it up, and shoot it down. I immediately feel the results. It wakes me up like an espresso shot. I feel more awake within moments after drinking this stuff. I strongly recommend mixing it with apple juice over water or any other juice. I really truly love green superfood powder and I know it helps my body to be in its very best condition. I swear I'll be taking this stuff until I die… if I ever do!

If you're one of those close-minded people who won't even try this green superfood powder, then at least have a daily multivitamin and extra vitamin C. Even if they are all-natural *Flintstones* chewable vitamins that you would take with your kids. They are good for you, plus you will be setting a good example for your children. Sometimes when I have a sweet tooth, I go in my cupboard and get a chewable vitamin C or a few chewable multivitamins. I eat those and drink cold water right after. That always does the trick.

Who still drinks tap water?

Don't drink tap water! I know some people think that the tap water in their area is good to drink. Wrong! Every city in the world has impurities in their tap water that come from industrial pollutants and chemicals such as chlorine that are added to the water to kill bacteria. They may kill the bacteria, which is good, however you are still drinking chlorine, which is a toxin. Filtered water takes out the chlorine, lead, fluoride, mercury, benzene, and other toxic chemicals in tap water that are harmful to your body. So drink any type of water that is filtered. Heck... boil water and let it cool if you have to. (This kills all the bacteria and removes all the chemicals.) Drink filtered water whether it's from the *Arrowhead* or *Sparkletts* deliveryman, or bottled water from the store. One simple and cheap filter that I recommend is a *Brita*. This little guy is just a water pitcher with a filter on top that you just fill up from the sink. Like any water filter, you just have to change the filter once in a while. You can get a *Brita* pitcher online or at any local drugstore. If you have a refrigerator that has filtered water, that works too. If it comes out too slow, it just means that you need to replace the filter. Other types of filters that are good are the ones that attach under your kitchen sink and have a spout that comes out over the sink. I have a good one of these from *Aquasana* (www.aquasana.com) and I drank water from it for years. (They also make shower filters that I have on every shower in the house.) Currently – because I am kind of extreme when it comes to water – I have a $2,000 water ionizer attached to my kitchen sink for my drinking water in order to have the purest, highest anti-oxidant, and alkaline water I can. If you can afford it, get one of these or go on their website, and compare and contrast for yourself (www.tyentusa.com). But the bottom line is, just drink any kind of filtered water.

THE RECAP

- First and foremost, do a colon/bowel cleanse (every year)
- Follow up with a liver/gallbladder cleanse (every 3 years)
- End with a kidney cleanse (every 3 years)
- Drink lots of water and eat plenty of fruits, vegetables, and fiber to flush toxins out of your body on a daily basis
- Stay away from processed and unnatural foods
- Always read the ingredients part of the nutrition facts on the foods you eat and avoid foods with artificial flavors and/or colors, preservatives, monosodium glutamate (MSG), and pretty much anything you can't pronounce
- The smaller the number of ingredients, the healthier the food
- Get a natural deodorant (*Aloe & Almonds* by Alvera on www.vitacost.com)
- Stay away from chemical, artificial sweeteners
- Switch to stevia, a natural calorie-free sweetener (carry packets with you)
- Look to get yourself off unnecessary prescriptions (consult your physician)
- Have green superfood powder everyday
- Drink any kind of filtered water instead of tap water

CONCLUSION

If someone came up to me saying, "I'm sick and tired of looking so good and lean, I'm sick and tired of fitting into my clothes so well and getting compliments from people, I'm sick and tired of having a lot of energy and inspiring people to lose weight and live a healthier lifestyle. And all that is happening because of your book *How to Lose Weight in Your Sleep*! Now I want to be FAT!" Here is what I would say to this person in my new book *How to Gain Weight in Your Sleep*.

Wake up every morning and do not eat breakfast. Drink tons of coffee and don't drink water, so you will be totally dehydrated and will also have a huge appetite for later. Move around really slowly, using as little energy as possible. When it's lunchtime, eat a huge meal. A super-sized fast food meal with a diet soda would be the best option. Eat so much that you feel so full and so tired that, when you go back to work, you have to have more coffee, which will dehydrate you even more. Make sure you put lots of artificial sweeteners in it, because they help increase your appetite and preserve your fat. After work, don't ever even think about working out, because you wouldn't want to put on any lean muscle from weights (which would only burn more calories), let alone burn off any of that precious fat from doing cardio. At home, sit around and see if you can create more unresolved issues with people, because the more grudges you hold, the more fat you will hold. Then when it gets near bedtime, eat one more gigantic meal and then go straight to bed. But before you go to sleep, do a quick visualization, imagining yourself really fat. And don't ever think about doing a cleanse, because you want all the food and toxins to accumulate in your body in order to slow down your metabolism as much as possible. These are the keys on how to gain weight in your sleep.

Now this silly and absurd example would never happen because people are always going to want to lose weight in order to feel good and look their best. In this book, I have exhausted all my information and all my secrets on how to lose weight in your sleep, so that everybody can do it. This material works and will always work as long as we have human bodies. This is the best way to have your best body, even a thousand years from now. So I pass this information along to you. Use it. It will work wonders for you as long as you follow it. Like anything in the beginning, it's going to be an adjustment. But remember, *it's not a diet, it's a lifestyle change.* It may take one to two weeks for you and your body to adapt and get used to this new lifestyle. You've been used to eating a certain way for a long time now, so it's going to take some time to get used to this new way of doing things. Be as consistent as you can, but it's really important not to beat yourself up if you slip up. If you miss a workout that you planned to do or if you eat over your amount of calories, it's okay. You're adjusting to everything, so forgive yourself and keep moving forward with it. As you start to implement this new lifestyle, you'll see how your body is going to incredibly transform without that much effort. You will look great, feel great, have more energy, and you will inspire others. All that from losing weight in your sleep. Sweet dreams...

QUICK REFERENCE GUIDE

Now you have read the book, you were given the details, and this part is just an overall recap that you can re-read and refer to at anytime.

Stop giving your body a reason to store fat

Our body only stores fat because we've given it a reason to do so. Fat isn't bad, and your body has done great by storing it. It has been very effective based on the circumstances and environment you have put it in. Now, if you want to stop giving your body a reason to store fat, you must change the circumstances your body's been in. In other words, you have to do things different and adopt a new lifestyle.

Eat every 3 hours

We came into this world as babies who were hungry and were fed every 3 hours. This shows us how the human body wants to receive nutrients and how to have a metabolism functioning optimally. If you go hours and hours without eating, your body is not getting any nutrients so it thinks it is starving, and it will slow its metabolism down and go into fat storage mode. So when you do eat, your body is going to store as much as it can as fat. Remember, fat is stored energy for later. So going long periods of time without eating is exactly how you become fat. Instead, eat every 3 hours so your body won't have a reason to store fat.

Don't be a sumo

Sumo wrestlers eat one meal a day. One huge meal! So the opposite of that is to eat like we did as babies and little kids, small meals every 3 hours. Why do you think kids have so much energy? Because their blood sugar levels are always stable. If you eat small meals every 3 hours, your body will constantly get fuel right when it needs it. So if you don't want to look like a sumo, then don't eat like a sumo.

Be hungry every 3 hours

You don't just want to eat every 3 hours, you want to be hungry every 3 hours. The key is to eat a small amount (two cupped hands or less) so that you will be hungry 3 hours later. As a guide, you want your stomach to lightly growl or feel a warm sensation in your stomach like it's about to growl, every 3 hours. This will naturally alert you when it's time to eat. If this doesn't happen 3 hours after eating, you simply ate too much at your previous meal, and if it happens before 3 hours, you ate too little. Now you just need to adjust.

You may just be thirsty not hungry

Be aware that the feeling of thirst is often mistaken for being hungry. So you may think that you are hungry, when in fact you are really dehydrated. If you feel that you might be hungry but your stomach is not growling or feeling like it's about to growl, then you are just thirsty. So drink lots of water. Water is good for us, it detoxifies the body and it is a natural appetite suppressant.

Always have clear pee

Use the pee test to see if you are dehydrated. The more yellow it is, the more dehydrated you are. So drink plenty of water to always have clear pee. And yes, you will pee more, but there's nothing wrong with that because you will be constantly keeping your cells hydrated and flushing out harmful toxins, which will relieve stress on your liver and kidneys, and keep you looking younger.

Your calorie formula

In order to find how many calories you should be eating to be at your dream weight, take the weight you want to weigh (not your current weight), then multiply by 12, and divide that number by 5. That's approximately how many calories you should be eating every 3 hours to be at your dream weight. You can go under that amount if you want, just don't go over it.

Right before it's time to eat... sleep

Don't eat 3 hours before you go to bed. This is key in order to burn fat in your sleep. When it's time to go to bed, your body will be ready to eat again because you've been eating every 3 hours throughout the day and it's been 3 hours since your last meal. But instead of eating again, you're going to drink water and go to bed. See, your body is expecting to get energy from food, but since there's no food coming, it's going to use and burn its own fat for its next meal.

Hurray for the cheat day

You're going to give yourself a cheat day once a week because it's important to know that you can still eat whatever and however you want. It reminds you that this is not a diet, but a lifestyle change, and you're allowed to cheat as much or as little as you like once a week.

Only work out every other day

Work up to doing 30 minutes of weight training and 30 minutes of any type of cardio that gets your heart rate up. One hour every other day amounts to 3.5 hours out of a 168-hour week, so it's really not much at all. If you can, join a gym. At the gym, use weights or weight machines, and use different types of cardio machines. When you find it hard to have a conversation during cardio, it means you are in your fat burning zone. If you don't want to join a gym, yoga classes are great. If that's still out of the question, you can always do any exercise video you like at home or my 3-day Soup Can Workout. Afterwards you can walk the dog fast or go on a brisk walk with the intention to get your heart rate up. Always remember to stretch in between weight training sets and after cardio.

Visualize what you want to look like right before you sleep

Right when you lay your head on the pillow, imagine that you already are at your dream weight. Picture yourself looking in the mirror, seeing and feeling how thin you are. Do it every night for 30 seconds, smiling and feeling good.

Identify any irrational beliefs or misunderstandings you may have

Determine if you have any subconscious beliefs that are irrational. Your powerful mind might still be holding on to false beliefs. As kids, we were sponges, but parents or authoritative figures didn't know what they were doing or saying half of the time. So forgive yourself for buying into any irrational beliefs, tell yourself what the real truth is, and move on. You'll find that identifying irrational beliefs or misunderstandings you may have from childhood will take away their power, and you as well as your body will start behaving in a rational way.

Resolve unresolved issues

Handle any unresolved issues you may have with other people. It could be blocking you from losing weight. Take the higher road and contact that person. It's time. By letting the ego go, your body will let the fat go.

Cleanse the body

Doing a cleanse will flush toxins out of your body so that your organs can do their job optimally, which will allow your metabolism to work even faster. And that's exactly what you want in order to burn fat in your sleep. Start with a colon/bowel cleanse, then later do a liver/gallbladder cleanse, and last do a kidney cleanse. It's recommended to do a simple colon/bowel cleanse once a year, and you only need to do a liver/gallbladder and kidney cleanse every three years.

Keep the toxins out

You have to prevent toxins from going into your body in order to continue to have a fast metabolism. Avoid processed foods, foods with artificial flavors, colors, or preservatives. Stay away from artificial sweeteners. They are chemicals that are not only bad for your health, but also increase your appetite, make you gain weight, and preserve your fat. Use unprocessed brown sugar, agave nectar, honey, or better yet get stevia. Look at the ingredients in the foods you eat. If you can't pronounce it, then it's probably not good for you. The least amount of ingredients the product has, the better.

MEAL PLANS: HOME-PREPARED

I've provided the calories for each food so feel free to mix up and substitute different foods for each other as well as different meals for one another. Some meals are slightly over or slightly under the specific calorie number. This is okay as long as the average meal that day is right at or under your calorie number.

WOMEN

Dream weight: 120 pounds

Calories per meal: about 290 calories or less

MONDAY

MEAL 1 - Oatmeal

½ cup apple juice (60cal)

1 scoop green superfood powder (50cal)

1 packet cinnamon instant oatmeal (170cal)

= 280cal

MEAL 2 - Fruit snack

1 mango (200cal)

2 kiwis (80cal)

= 280cal

MEAL 3 - Quinoa salad

¾ cup cooked quinoa (165cal)

1 cooked beet (35cal)

3 cooked carrots (90cal)

= 290cal

MEAL 4 - Bar & fruit

½ apple (45cal)

1 Cliff bar White Chocolate Macadamia (250cal)

= 295cal

MEAL 5 - Chicken with rice

½ chicken breast (140cal)

½ cup cooked brown rice (110cal)

½ cup green beans (15cal)

¼ cup applesauce (25cal)

= 290cal

TUESDAY

MEAL 1 - Corn flakes

1 cup orange juice (115cal)

1 cup corn flakes (100cal)

¾ cup milk, 1 % milkfat (75cal)

= 290cal

MEAL 2 - Crackers & banana

1 banana (105cal)

6 graham crackers (180cal)

= 285cal

MEAL 3 - Tuna sandwich

1 slice whole wheat bread (70cal)

3oz white tuna, canned in water (110cal)

1 tbsp mayonnaise, reduced fat (50cal)

1 peach (60cal)

= 290cal

MEAL 4 - Rice cakes & peanut butter

2 tbsp peanut butter (190cal)

3 plain rice cakes (105cal)

= 295cal

MEAL 5 - Egg whites & toast

4 egg whites (60cal)

1 cup spinach (5cal)

1 slice whole wheat bread (70cal)

1 tsp butter (35cal)

1 tbsp jam (55cal)

1 orange (60cal)

= 280cal

WEDNESDAY

MEAL 1 - Yogurt & berries

½ cup apple juice (60cal)

1 scoop green superfood powder (50cal)

½ cup plain yogurt, low fat (75cal)

¾ cup blueberries (60cal)

¾ cup strawberries (35cal)

= 280cal

MEAL 2 - Bar & fruit

1 apple (95cal)

1 Power Crunch bar Peanut Butter fudge (200cal)

= 295cal

MEAL 3 - Quinoa salad

½ cup cooked quinoa (110cal)

½ cup chickpeas (135cal)

2 cups arugula (10cal)

1 cup cherry tomatoes (25cal)

1 tbsp balsamic (15cal)

= 295cal

MEAL 4 - Hummus & pita

½ pita bread (85cal)

1/3 cup hummus (135cal)

2 clementines (70cal)

= 290cal

MEAL 5 - Sardines with pasta

4 sardines, canned in oil (100cal)

¾ cup cooked whole wheat pasta (130cal)

¼ cup tomato sauce (15cal)

½ cup cherries (40cal)

= 285cal

THURSDAY

MEAL 1 - Yogurt parfait

1 cup orange juice (115cal)

½ cup plain yogurt, low fat (75cal)

2 tbsp granola (75cal)

2 apricots (30cal)

= 295cal

MEAL 2 - Graham crackers with peanut butter

1 banana (105cal)

3 graham crackers (90cal)

1 tbsp almond butter (100cal)

= 295cal

MEAL 3 - Turkey sandwich

2 slices whole wheat bread (140cal)

3 slices turkey lunch meat (90cal)

1 tomato (10cal)

1 cup lettuce (5cal)

1 tbsp mayonnaise, reduced fat (50cal)

= 295cal

MEAL 4 - Mango-pineapple smoothie

1 cup milk, 1% milkfat (100cal)

1 cup pineapple chunks (80cal)

1 cup mango pieces (100cal)

= 280cal

MEAL 5 - Scrambled eggs with mushrooms

5 egg whites (75cal)

2 cups sliced mushrooms (30cal)

2 tbsp parmesan (55cal)

2 cups spinach (10cal)

1 tbsp balsamic vinegar (15cal)

1 apple, slices (95cal)

= 280cal

FRIDAY

MEAL 1 - Peanut butter toast

½ cup apple juice (60cal)

1 scoop green superfood powder (50cal)

1 slice whole wheat bread (70cal)

1 tbsp peanut butter (95cal)

= 275cal

MEAL 2 - Granola yogurt parfait

1 cup plain yogurt, low fat (150cal)

3 tbsp granola (110cal)

½ cup raspberries (30cal)

= 290cal

MEAL 3 - Salmon with pasta

2oz salmon (100cal)

1 cup cooked whole wheat pasta (175cal)

¼ cup tomato sauce (15cal)

= 290cal

MEAL 4 - Guacamole & tortilla chips

½ avocado, mashed (160cal)

13 blue corn tortilla chips (130cal)

= 290cal

MEAL 5 - Turkey

3oz ground turkey (130cal)

½ cooked potato (60cal)

1 cooked carrot (30cal)

1 ½ cup strawberries, whole (75cal)

= 295cal

SATURDAY

MEAL 1 - Yogurt flakes

1 cup orange juice (115cal)

½ cup plain yogurt, low fat (75cal)

¾ cup bran flakes (75cal)

= 285cal

MEAL 2 - Banana-strawberry smoothie

1 cup milk, 1% milkfat (100cal)

1 banana (105cal)

1 ½ cups strawberries (75cal)

= 280cal

MEAL 3 - Tortilla wrap

1 corn tortilla (50cal)

½ cup black beans (115cal)

¼ cup cheddar cheese, low fat (50cal)

½ cup sweet corn (60cal)

1 tomato (10cal)

= 285cal

MEAL 4 - Peanut butter and jelly

1 slice whole wheat bread (70cal)

1 tbsp peanut butter (95cal)

2 tbsp jam (110cal)

= 275cal

MEAL 5 - Couscous salad

½ cup cooked couscous (90cal)

½ English cucumber (20cal)

½ cup cherry tomatoes (10cal)

2 tbsp crumbled feta (50cal)

¼ onion (15cal)

1 apple, slices (95cal)

= 280cal

SUNDAY

MEAL 1 - Scrambled eggs with parmesan

½ cup apple juice (60cal)

1 scoop green superfood powder (50cal)

1 whole egg (70cal)

3 egg whites (45cal)

2 tbsp parmesan (55cal)

= 280cal

MEAL 2 - Almond butter & banana toast

1 slice whole wheat bread (70cal)

1 tbsp almond butter (100cal)

1 banana, sliced (105cal)

¼ cup blueberries (20cal)

= 295cal

MEAL 3 - Chicken with rice

3oz ground chicken (160cal)

½ cup cooked brown rice (110cal)

½ cup broccoli (15cal)

= 285cal

MEAL 4 - Nut & fruit snack

¼ cup almonds (205cal)

1 cup cherries (85cal)

= 290cal

MEAL 5 - Halibut with asparagus

5oz halibut filet (150cal)

1 tsp butter (35cal)

10 asparagus spears (50cal)

1 orange (60cal)

= 295cal

MEN

Dream weight: 170 pounds
Calories per meal: about 410 calories or less

MONDAY

MEAL 1 - Oatmeal

½ cup apple juice (60cal)
1 scoop green superfood powder (50cal)
1 packet cinnamon instant oatmeal (170cal)
¼ cup raisins (120cal)
= 400cal

MEAL 2 - Rice cakes & peanut butter

4 plain rice cakes (140cal)
2 tbsp peanut butter (190cal)
1 orange (60cal)
= 390cal

MEAL 3 - Tuna sandwich

2 slices whole wheat bread (140cal)
6oz tuna, canned in water (220cal)
1 cup romaine lettuce (5cal)
1 tbsp mayonnaise, reduced fat (50cal)
= 415cal

MEAL 4 - Bar & fruit

1 Promax bar Nutty Butter Crisp (300cal)
1 banana (105cal)
= 405cal

MEAL 5 - Chicken with rice

4oz chicken breast (185cal)

½ cup cooked brown rice (110cal)

1 zucchini (30cal)

1 apple (95cal)

= 420cal

TUESDAY

MEAL 1 - Corn flakes

½ cup orange juice (60cal)

2 cups corn flakes (200cal)

1 ½ cup milk, 1% milkfat (150cal)

= 410cal

MEAL 2 - Crackers & cottage cheese

25 wheat crackers (225cal)

½ cup cottage cheese, 1% milkfat (80cal)

1 apple (95cal)

= 400cal

MEAL 3 - Yogurt with berries & almonds

1 cup plain yogurt, low fat (150cal)

½ cup blueberries (40cal)

¼ cup almonds (205cal)

= 395cal

MEAL 4 - Bar

MET-Rx bar Supreme Cookie Crunch (410cal)

= 410cal

MEAL 5 - Beef steak with rice

3oz top sirloin beef steak (180cal)

½ cup cooked brown rice (110cal)

1 cup steamed broccoli (30cal)

2 tbsp steak sauce (30cal)

1 orange, slices (60cal)

= 410cal

WEDNESDAY

MEAL 1 - Yogurt & granola

½ cup apple juice (60cal)

1 scoop green superfood powder (50cal)

1 cup plain yogurt, low fat (150cal)

¼ cup granola (150cal)

= 410cal

MEAL 2 - Bars

2 Power Crunch bars Peanut Butter Crème (400cal)

= 400cal

MEAL 3 - Quinoa salad

½ cup cooked quinoa (110cal)

6oz ground turkey (260cal)

2 cups arugula (10cal)

½ cup cherry tomatoes (25cal)

1 tbsp balsamic vinegar (15cal)

= 420cal

MEAL 4 - Hummus & pita

1 pita bread (170cal)

½ cup hummus (200cal)

1 tbsp crumbled feta (25cal)

= 395cal

MEAL 5 - Salmon with rice

4oz salmon (200cal)

½ cup cooked brown rice (110cal)

1 cup grapes (100cal)

= 410cal

THURSDAY

MEAL 1 - Egg whites & toast

6 egg whites (90cal)

1 cup spinach (5cal)

2 slices whole wheat bread (140cal)

2 tbsp strawberry (110cal)

½ cup orange juice (60cal)

= 405cal

MEAL 2 - Banana & peanut butter

1 banana (105cal)

2 tbsp peanut butter (190cal)

1 cup orange juice (115cal)

= 410cal

MEAL 3 - Turkey sandwich

2 slices whole wheat bread (140cal)

5 slices turkey lunch meat (150cal)

1 tomato (10cal)

1 cup romaine lettuce (5cal)

2 tbsp mayonnaise, reduced fat (100cal)

= 405cal

MEAL 4 - Pineapple-mango protein shake
1 cup milk, 1% milkfat (100cal)

1 ¼ cup pineapple chunks (100cal)

1 ¼ cup mango pieces (125cal)

1 scoop MRM vanilla protein powder (85cal)

= 410cal

MEAL 5 - Sardines with pasta
8 sardines, canned in oil (200cal)

½ cup cooked whole wheat pasta (85cal)

½ cup tomato sauce (30cal)

1 apple (95cal)

= 410cal

FRIDAY

MEAL 1 - Peanut butter & jelly toast
½ cup apple juice (60cal)

1 scoop green superfood powder (50cal)

2 slices whole wheat bread (140cal)

1 tbsp peanut butter (95cal)

1 tbsp jam (55cal)

= 400cal

MEAL 2 - Bar & fruit
1 Clif bar White Chocolate Macadamia (250cal)

1 banana (105cal)

½ cup orange juice (60cal)

= 415cal

MEAL 3 - Chicken salad

1 chicken breast (280cal)

4 cups romaine lettuce (20cal)

1 tbsp walnuts (50cal)

1 cup cherry tomatoes (25cal)

2 tbsp balsamic vinegar (30cal)

= 405cal

MEAL 4 - Granola & fruit

1 cup plain yogurt, low fat (150cal)

¼ cup granola (150cal)

1 pear (100cal)

= 400cal

MEAL 5 - Eggs with ham

1 whole egg (70cal)

4 egg whites (60cal)

½ cup sliced mushrooms (5cal)

2 tbsp parmesan (55cal)

2 slices ham (80cal)

1 slice whole wheat bread (70cal)

1 tbsp jam (55cal)

= 405cal

SATURDAY

MEAL 1 - Yogurt flakes

½ cup apple juice (60cal)

1 scoop green superfood powder (50cal)

1 cup plain yogurt, low fat (150cal)

1 cup bran flakes (100cal)

1 tbsp pecan halves (45cal)

= 405cal

MEAL 2 - Banana-strawberry protein shake

1 cup milk, 1% milkfat (100cal)

1 banana (105cal)

2 ½ cups strawberries (125cal)

1 scoop MRM chocolate protein powder (85cal)

= 415cal

MEAL 3 - Chicken tortilla wrap

1 corn tortilla (50cal)

½ cup black beans (115cal)

¼ cup cheddar cheese, low fat (50cal)

¼ cup sweet corn (30cal)

2 tomatoes (20cal)

½ chicken breast (140cal)

= 405cal

MEAL 4 - Peanut butter & jelly with fruit

2 slices whole wheat bread (140cal)

1 tbsp peanut butter (95cal)

1 tbsp jam (55cal)

1 banana (105cal)

= 395cal

MEAL 5 - Turkey salad

3oz ground turkey (130cal)

½ cup cooked couscous (90cal)

1 English cucumber (45cal)

½ cup cherry tomatoes (10cal)

¼ cup crumbled feta (100cal)

¼ onion

1 tbsp balsamic vinegar

= 410cal

SUNDAY

MEAL 1 - Eggs with tomatoes

½ cup apple juice (60cal)

1 scoop green superfood powder (50cal)

1 whole egg (70cal)

5 egg whites (75cal)

1 cup cherry tomatoes (25cal)

¼ cup parmesan (110cal)

= 390cal

MEAL 2 - Bar

2 Balance bars Double Chocolate Brownie (400cal)

= 400cal

MEAL 3 - Cottage cheese & tortilla chips

¾ cup cottage cheese, 1% milkfat (120cal)

20 blue corn tortilla chips (200cal)

1 apple (95cal)

= 415cal

MEAL 4 - Peanut butter-banana protein shake

1 cup milk, 1% milkfat (100cal)

1 tbsp peanut butter (95cal)

1 banana (105cal)

1 scoop chocolate protein powder (110cal)

= 410cal

MEAL 5 - Halibut fillet

3oz halibut fillet (90cal)

½ cup brown rice (110cal)

1 tbsp butter (100cal)

4 asparagus (20cal)

1 cup cherries (85cal)

= 405cal

MEAL PLANS: ON-THE-GO

MEAL REPLACEMENT BARS

Food bars have come a long way over the years and many of them not only don't taste like cardboard, but are delicious and nutritious. You can buy them at almost any gas station, liquor store, drugstore, or grocery store. These are a few I recommend that taste good and are all-natural. I personally have at least one or two of these every day either by themselves or with a piece of fruit.

Brand name	Calorie range
Balance	200-210
CarbRite Diet	190-200
Clif	230-250
Clif Builder's	270-280
Greens Plus Whey Krisp	210
Larabar	190-240
Lenny & Larry's Muscle Brownie	170
Luna	170-190
MET-Rx, Big 100	370-430

Perfect Foods	305-310
Perfect Foods Lite	200
Power Crunch	200-210
Promax	270-300
Promax, LS (Low Sugar)	220-240
PowerBar, Protein Plus	270-360
PowerBar, Harvest	240-250
Think Thin, High Protein Bars	200-240
Quest	160-210
Zone Perfect	180-210

FAST FOOD

I am not an advocate of fast food. However, in certain situations it may be the most convenient option for you. The following is to show you that you can still stay in your calorie range even if you had to have fast food once in a great while.

MCDONALD'S

Women

MEAL 1
Egg McMuffin (300cal)

MEAL 2
Fruit & Walnuts (210cal)

MEAL 3
Cheeseburger (300cal)

MEAL 4
Small McCafé Mango Pineapple Real Fruit Smoothie (220cal)

MEAL 5
Ranch Snack Wrap, Grilled (270cal)

MCDONALD'S

Men

MEAL 1
Sausage McMuffin (370cal)

MEAL 2
Honey Mustard Snack Wrap, Grilled (250cal)
Fruit 'N Yogurt Parfait (150cal)
= 400cal

MEAL 3
McDouble (390cal)

MEAL 4
Small McCafé Strawberry Banana Real Fruit Smoothie (210cal)
4 Chicken McNuggets (190cal)
= 400cal

MEAL 5
Filet-O-Fish (380cal)
Apple slices (15cal)
= 395cal

BURGER KING

Women

MEAL 1
Croissan'wich, Egg & Cheese (280cal)

MEAL 2
2 Homestyle Chicken Strips (240cal)
Apple slices (30cal)
= 270cal

MEAL 3
Side of Caesar Salad & Dressing (280cal)

MEAL 4
4 Mozzarella Sticks (280cal)

MEAL 5
6 Chicken Nuggets (290cal)

BURGER KING

Men

MEAL 1
Breakfast Muffin Sandwich, Sausage, Egg & Cheese (390cal)

MEAL 2
Honey Mustard Crispy Chicken Wrap (390cal)

MEAL 3
Original Chicken Sandwich, without mayonnaise (420cal)

MEAL 4
Double Cheeseburger (370cal)
Apple slices (30cal)
= 400cal

MEAL 5
Premium Alaskan Fish Sandwich, without tartar sauce (410cal)

WENDY'S

Women

MEAL 1
Sausage & Egg Burrito (270cal)

MEAL 2
5 Chicken Nuggets (220cal)
Honey Mustard Nugget Sauce (80cal)
= 300cal

MEAL 3
Jr. Cheeseburger (290cal)

MEAL 4
Half-Size Spicy Chicken Caesar Salad (250cal)
Fat Free French Dressing (40cal)
= 290cal

MEAL 5
Grilled Chicken Go Wrap (260cal)

WENDY'S

Men

MEAL 1
Sausage & Cheese Muffin (430cal)

MEAL 2
Apple Pecan Chicken Salad (350cal)
Pomegranate Vinaigrette Dressing (60cal)
= 410cal

MEAL 3
Jr. Bacon Cheeseburger (400cal)

MEAL 4
Ultimate Chicken Grill Sandwich (390cal)

MEAL 5
Double Stack Cheeseburger (400cal)

KFC

Women

MEAL 1
2 Crispy Strips (260cal)
Sweet & Sour Dipping Sauce Cup (45cal)
= 305cal

MEAL 2
Side of Macaroni & Cheese (160cal)
Side of Sweet Kernel Corn (100cal)
Side of Green Beans (25cal)
= 285cal

MEAL 3
Biscuit (180cal)
Mashed Potatoes with Gravy (120cal)
= 300cal

MEAL 4
Snacker with Crispy Strip Ultimate Cheese Sandwich (280cal)

MEAL 5
Grilled Chicken Breast (220cal)
3" Corn on the Cob (70cal)
= 290cal

KFC

Men

MEAL 1
Popcorn Chicken Individual (400cal)

MEAL 2
Drumstick Value Box (400cal)

MEAL 3
Snacker Honey BBQ Sandwich (210cal)
Side of BBQ Baked Beans (210cal)
= 420

MEAL 4
Crispy Chicken BLT Salad (360cal)
Hidden Valley The Original Ranch Fat Free Dressing (35cal)
= 395

MEAL 5
Grilled Chicken Breast (220cal)
Side of Mashed Potatoes with Gravy (120cal)
Side of 3" Corn on the Cob (70cal)
= 380

SUBWAY

Unless indicated, the below items are without cheese, mayonnaise, or oil & vinegar. Mustard and veggies only.

Women

MEAL 1
Breakfast BMT Melt on 3" Flatbread (250cal)

MEAL 2
6" Veggie Delite (230cal)
Apple slices (35cal)
= 265cal

MEAL 3
6" Turkey Breast on 9-Grain Wheat Bread (280cal)

MEAL 4
Grilled Chicken Salad (130cal)
Baby Spinach with Fat Free Italian Dressing (35cal)
Yogurt Parfait Granola (130cal)
= 295cal

MEAL 5
6" Black Forest Ham on 9-Grain Wheat Bread (290cal)

SUBWAY

Men

MEAL 1
Egg & Cheese with Ham Omelet on 6" Flatbread (400cal)

MEAL 2
6" Veggie Delite on 9-Grain Wheat Bread (230cal)
Yogurt Parfait with Granola (160cal)
= 390cal

MEAL 3
6" Turkey Breast & Black Forest Ham on 9-Grain Wheat Bread (280cal)
Baked Lay's (130cal)
= 410cal

MEAL 4
Sweet Onion Chicken Teriyaki Salad with Oil & Vinegar Dressing (390cal)

MEAL 5
6" Italian BMT on 9-Grain Wheat Bread (410cal)

TACO BELL

Women

MEAL 1
Cinnabon Delights (220cal)

MEAL 2
Fresco Chicken Soft Taco (150cal)
Fresco Crunchy Taco (140cal)
= 290cal

MEAL 3
MexiMelt (270cal)

MEAL 4
Toastada (250cal)

MEAL 5
Gordita Supreme Beef (300cal)

TACO BELL

Men

MEAL 1
Sausage & Egg Wrap (360cal)

MEAL 2
Black Bean Burrito (410cal)

MEAL 3
Cheesy Nachos (270cal)
Fresco Grilled Steak Soft Taco (150cal)
= 420cal

MEAL 4
Crunchy Taco Supreme (200cal)
Side of Black Beans & Rice (200cal)
= 400cal

MEAL 5
Gordita Chicken Supreme (270cal)
Fresco Crunchy Taco (140cal)
= 410cal

CARL'S JUNIOR / HARDEE'S

Women

MEAL 1
Sourdough Breakfast Sandwich with Ham & Swiss Cheese only (300cal)

MEAL 2
3 Hand Breaded Chicken Tenders (260cal)

MEAL 3
Original Grilled Chicken Salad (280cal)
Low Fat Balsamic Vinaigrette Dressing (35cal)
= 315cal

MEAL 4
Kid's Hamburger (280cal)

MEAL 5
Honey Mustard Hand Breaded Chicken Tender Wrapper (290cal)

CARL'S JUNIOR / HARDEE'S

Men

MEAL 1
Ham Biscuit with Swiss Cheese (380cal)

MEAL 2
9 Chicken Stars (390cal)

MEAL 3
Turkey Burger, no mayonnaise (380cal)

MEAL 4
Famous Star, no cheese, mustard and ketchup instead of mayonnaise or special sauce (420cal)

MEAL 5
Charbroiled BBQ Chicken Sandwich (390cal)

JACK IN THE BOX

Women

MEAL 1
Breakfast Jack (280cal)

MEAL 2
3 Mozzarella Cheese Sticks (280cal)

MEAL 3
Chicken Fajita Pita made with Whole Grain, no cheese (230cal)
1 Egg Roll (60cal)
= 290cal

MEAL 4
16 oz Strawberry Banana Smoothie (290cal)

MEAL 5
Hamburger (290cal)

JACK IN THE BOX

Men

MEAL 1
Sourdough Breakfast Sandwich (410cal)

MEAL 2
Pita Snack Steak (350cal)
Fruit Cup (50cal)
= 400cal

MEAL 3
Hamburger Delux with Cheese (410cal)

MEAL 4
Chicken Sandwich (410cal)

MEAL 5
Jr. Bacon Cheeseburger (390cal)

STARBUCKS

Women

MEAL 1
Spinach & Feta Breakfast Wrap (290cal)

MEAL 2
Strawberry Blueberry Yogurt Parfait (290cal)

MEAL 3
Chipotle Chicken Wrap Bistro Box (290cal)

MEAL 4
Chocolate Croissant (300cal)

MEAL 5
Chicken Hummus Bistro Box (260cal)

STARBUCKS

Men

MEAL 1
Apple Bran Muffin (350cal)

MEAL 2
Chicken Santa Fe Panini (400cal)

MEAL 3
Turkey & Swiss Sandwich (390cal)

MEAL 4
Tuna Salad Bistro Box (380cal)

MEAL 5
Tarragon Chicken Salad Sandwich (420cal)

CALORIE GUIDE

The calorie numbers given here are based on the USDA
National Nutrient Database for Standard Reference
http://ndb.nal.usda.gov/ndb/foods/list
The number of calories in foods can vary from one brand to
another, so the purpose of this guide is only to give you the
average number of calories in foods so you get an idea. The
numbers are rounded off to make it easier for you to use.

Vegetables

	Serving size	Calories
Artichoke	1 medium	60
Arugula	1 cup	5
Asparagus	1 extra-large	5
Beet	1	35
Broccoli	1 cup, chopped	30
Brussels sprouts	5	40
Cabbage	1 cup, shredded	15
Carrots	1 large	30

Cauliflower	1 cup, chopped	30
Celery	1 medium stalk	5
Corn, sweet	1 cup kernels	125
Cucumber, English	1, with peel	45
Eggplant	1, unpeeled	130
Endive	1 head	85
Fennel	1 bulb	70
Green beans	1 cup, ½" pieces	30
Kale	1 cup, chopped	35
Leeks	1 bulb	55
Mushrooms, white	1 cup, slices	15
Onion	1 large	60
Parsnips	1 cup, slices	100
Peas, green	1 cup	115
Pepper, green	1 medium	25
Pepper, red	1 medium	35
Potatoes, red, white	1	120
Pumpkin	1 cup, cubes	30
Radishes	15 small	5
Romaine lettuce	1 cup, shredded	5
Spinach	1 cup	5
Squash, acorn	1 cup, cubes	55
Squash, butternut	1 cup, cubes	60
Sweet potato	1	110
Tomato, cherry	1 cup	25
Tomato, Italian, plum	1	10
Turnips	1 medium	35
Zucchini	1 medium	30

Fruits

	Serving size	Calories
Apple	1 medium	95
Apricot	1	15
Avocado	½	160
Banana	1 medium	105
Berries, blackberries	1 cup	60
Berries, blueberries	1 cup	80
Berries, raspberries	1 cup	60
Berries, strawberries	1 cup	50
Cherries	1 cup	85
Clementine	1	35
Grapefruit, pink, red, white	1	40
Grapes, red, green	1 cup	100
Kiwi	1	40
Lemon	1	15
Lime	1	20
Mango	1 cup pieces	100
Melon, cantaloupe	1 medium	190
Melon, honeydew	½ small	180
Nectarine	1 medium	60
Orange	1 medium	60
Papaya	1 small	70
Peach	1 medium	60
Pear	1 medium	100
Pineapple	1 cup, chunks	80
Plum	1	30

Raisins	¼ cup	120
Watermelon	1 cup, diced	45

Beans

Serving size ½ cup	Calories (uncooked)	Calories (cooked)
Black beans	330	115
Fava beans or broad beans	260	95
Garbanzo beans or chickpeas	365	135
Great Northern beans	310	105
Kidney beans	305	110
Lima beans	300	110
Mung beans	360	110
Navy beans	350	130
Pinto beans	335	120
White beans	335	125

Breads, grains, & pasta

	Serving size	Calories
Bagel, plain	1 small	190
Bread, pita, whole wheat	1 large	170
Bread, wheat	1 slice	80
Bread, whole wheat	1 slice	70
Couscous, cooked	½ cup	90

Couscous, uncooked	½ cup	325
Crackers, wheat	10 crackers	90
Flakes, bran, corn	1 cup	100
Graham crackers, honey, cinnamon	4 crackers	120
Granola	¼ cup	150
Oats, instant, cinnamon & spice	1 packet	170
Oats, regular and quick	½ cup	150
Pasta, cooked	1 cup	220
Pasta, uncooked	2 oz	210
Pasta, whole wheat, cooked	1 cup	175
Pasta, whole wheat, uncooked	2oz	200
Popcorn, air-popped	1 cup	30
Popcorn, unpopped kernels	¼ cup	210
Pretzels, plain	10 twists	230
Quinoa, cooked	½ cup	110
Quinoa, uncooked	½ cup	310
Rice cakes, brown rice, plain	1 cake	35
Rice, brown, cooked	½ cup	110
Rice, brown, uncooked	½ cup	345
Rice, white, cooked	½ cup	120
Rice, white, uncooked	½ cup	350
Rice, wild, cooked	½ cup	80
Rice, wild, uncooked	½ cup	285
Tortilla, corn	1 tortilla	50
Tortilla, flour	1 tortilla	90
Tortilla chips, yellow, plain	1 chip	12
Tortilla chips, blue, plain	1 chip	10

Meat, chicken, & poultry

As a guide, 3oz is about the size of a deck of playing cards.

	Serving size	Calories
Bacon, Canadian, grilled	3 slices	130
Beef, 95% extra lean, ground, cooked	1 patty	140
Beef, corned, cooked	3oz	210
Beef, flank, steak, trimmed fat, broiled	3oz	170
Beef, ground, 5% fat, patty, pan-broiled	3oz, 1 patty	140
Beef, top round, steak, trimmed fat, broiled	3oz	160
Beef, top sirloin, steak, trimmed fat, broiled	3oz	180
Chicken, breast, meat only, roasted	1 breast	280
Chicken, dark meat, meat only, roasted	3oz	170
Chicken, ground, crumbles, pan-browned	3oz	160
Ham, regular, sliced	1 slice	45
Pork, chops, boneless, lean, broiled	1	150
Turkey, breast, lunchmeat	1 slice	30
Turkey, dark meat, meat only, roasted	3oz	140
Turkey, ground, fat free, pan-broiled	3oz	130
Turkey, ground, fat free, patties, broiled	1 patty	120
Turkey, light meat, meat only, roasted	3oz	120
Turkey, sausage, breakfast links	2 links	130

Fish & seafood

	Serving size	Calories
Anchovy, canned in oil	8 anchovies	80
Cod, Atlantic, cooked	3oz	120
Crab cake	1	90
Crab, Alaskan king, leg, cooked	1	130
Crab, Alaskan king, made from surimi	3oz	80
Crab, blue, canned	1 can (6.5oz)	100
Halibut, Atlantic & Pacific, fillet, cooked	3oz	90
Lobster, Northern, cooked	3oz	80
Salmon, Atlantic, fillet, cooked	3oz	150
Sardine, Atlantic, canned in oil	4	100
Sea bass, cooked	1 fillet	125
Shrimp, cooked	12 large	80
Swordfish, cooked	3oz	150
Tuna, white, canned in oil	3oz	160
Tuna, white, canned in water	3oz	110

Dairy & eggs

	Serving size	Calories
Butter	1 tbsp	100
Cheese, cheddar, low fat, shredded	¼ cup	50
Cheese, cottage, 1% milkfat	¼ cup	40
Cheese, cream, low fat	¼ cup	120
Cheese, feta, crumbled	¼ cup	100

Cheese, monterey, low fat, shredded	¼ cup	90
Cheese, mozzarella, whole milk, shredded	¼ cup	80
Cheese, parmesan, grated	¼ cup	110
Cheese, ricotta, whole milk	¼ cup	110
Cheese, Swiss, low fat, shredded	¼ cup	50
Egg white	1 large	15
Egg, whole	1 large	70
Milk, 1% milkfat	1 cup	100
Yogurt, plain, low fat	1 cup	150

Nuts, nut butters, & vegetable oils

	Serving size	Calories
Almond butter, plain	1 tbsp	100
Almonds	¼ cup	205
Brazil nuts	¼ cup	220
Cashew butter	1 tbsp	95
Cashews	¼ cup	200
Hazelnuts	¼ cup	210
Macadamia	¼ cup	240
Peanut butter	1 tbsp	95
Peanuts	¼ cup	215
Pecans	¼ cup	170
Pine nuts	¼ cup	230
Pistachio	¼ cup	175
Sesame butter or tahini	1 tbsp	95
Sesame seeds	¼ cup	205

Sunflower seed butter	1 tbsp	100
Sunflower seeds	¼ cup	185
Vegetable oil, canola	1 tbsp	125
Vegetable oil, coconut	1 tbsp	115
Vegetable oil, olive	1 tbsp	120
Walnuts	¼ cup	195

Others

	Serving size	Calories
Applesauce	½ cup	50
Cocoa powder, unsweetened	1 tbsp	10
Hummus	¼ cup	100
Jams & preserves	1 tbsp	55
Juice, apple, orange, unsweetened	1 cup	115
Juice, pineapple	1 cup	130
MRM protein powder, vanilla or chocolate	1 scoop	85
Seasoning, mayonnaise, reduced calorie	1 tbsp	50
Seasoning, balsamic vinegar	1 tbsp	15
Seasoning, Caesar	1 tbsp	80
Seasoning, mustard	1 tbsp	10
Seasoning, Ranch	1 tbsp	75
Seasoning, steak sauce	1 tbsp	15
Seasoning, sweet relish	1 tbsp	20
Seasoning, Thousand Island	1 tbsp	60
Seasoning, tomato sauce	¼ cup	15
Tofu, regular	½ cup	95

WEBSITES

For more info: www.howtoloseweightinyoursleep.com
Exercise video: www.youtube.com/sleepandloseweight
Dr. Schulze's cleanses: www.herbdoc.com
Kidney flush combo: www.rainforestnaturalpharmacy.com
Natural health remedies and detoxes: www.naturalcures.com
Alvera deodorant, bars, and more: www.vitacost.com
Drinking water filters and shower filters: www.aquasana.com
Drinking water ionizer: www.tyentusa.com
Spiritual Psychology: www.universityofsantamonica.edu

Follow the author on Twitter @_How2LoseWeight
Like *How to Lose Weight in Your Sleep* on Facebook